PRETEST®

Pharmacology

Notice

PRETEST®

Pharmacology

PreTest® Self-Assessment and Review

Eighth Edition

Senior Editor
Joseph R. DiPalma, M.D., D.Sc.
Emeritus Professor of Pharmacology and Medicine
Medical College of Pennsylvania and Hahnemann University
Philadelphia, Pennsylvania

Contributing Editors
Edward J. Barbieri, Ph.D.
Associate Professor of Pharmacology

G. John DiGregorio, M.D., Ph.D.
Professor of Pharmacology and Medicine

Andrew P. Ferko, Ph.D.
Associate Professor of Pharmacology

Medical College of Pennsylvania and Hahnemann University
Philadelphia, Pennsylvania

McGraw-Hill
Health Professions Division
PreTest® Series

New York St. Louis San Francisco Auckland
Bogotá Caracas Lisbon London Madrid
Mexico City Milan Montreal New Delhi
San Juan Singapore Sydney Tokyo Toronto

McGraw-Hill
A Division of The McGraw-Hill Companies

Pharmacology: PreTest® Self-Assessment and Review, Eighth Edition

1 2 3 4 5 6 7 8 9 0 DOCDOC 9 8 7 6 5

ISBN 0-07-052087-9

The editors were Gail Gavert and Bruce MacGregor.
The production supervisor was Gyl A. Favours.
R.R. Donnelley & Sons was printer and binder.
This book was set in Times Roman by Digitype.

Library of Congress Cataloging-in-Publication Data
Pharmacology : PreTest self-assessment and review / senior editor, Joseph R. DiPalma ; contributing editors, Edward J. Barbieri . . . [et al.]. — 8th ed.
p. cm.
Includes bibliographical references.
ISBN 0-07-052087-9 (pbk.)
1. Pharmacology—Examinations, questions, etc. I. DiPalma, Joseph R.
[DNLM: 1. Pharmacology—examination questions. QV 18.2 P536 1995]
RM301.13.P475 1996
615'.1'076—dc20
DNLM/DLC
for Library of Congress 95-3585

Contents

Contents

Introduction

Each *PreTest® Self-Assessment and Review* allows medical students to comprehensively and conveniently assess and review their knowledge of a particular basic science—in this instance, Pharmacology. The 500 questions parallel the format and degree of difficulty of the questions found in the United States Medical Licensing Examination (USMLE) Step 1. Practicing physicians who want to hone their skills before USMLE Step 3 or recertification may find this to be a good beginning in their review process.

Each question is accompanied by an answer, a paragraph explanation, and a specific page reference to an appropriate textbook. A bibliography listing sources can be found following the last chapter of this text.

Before each chapter, a list of key terms or classifications of drugs or both is included to aid review. In addition, suggestions for effective study and review have been added below.

The most effective method of using this book is to complete one chapter at a time. Prepare yourself for each chapter by reviewing from your notes and favorite text the drugs listed at the beginning of each section. You should concentrate especially on the prototype drugs, which are marked by an asterisk. Then proceed to indicate your answer by each question, allowing yourself not more than one minute for each question. In this way you will be approximating the time limits imposed by the Step.

After you finish going through the questions in the section, spend as much time as you need verifying your answers and carefully reading the explanations provided. Pay special attention to the explanations for the questions you answered incorrectly—but read *every* explanation. The editors of this material have designed the explanations to reinforce and supplement the information tested by the questions. If you feel you need further information about the material covered, consult and study the references indicated.

SUGGESTIONS FOR EFFECTIVE STUDY AND REVIEW

The study of pharmacology is not different from that of the other basic medical sciences. For most students pharmacology may seem more relevant than other subjects to the practice of clinical medicine. It has the advantage of coming last in the curriculum of basic sciences. Nevertheless, the disadvantage of pharmacology is the need to commit to memory an enormous number of names and facts about numerous drugs and furthermore to relate these to each other and to clinical medicine. Most students find it advantageous to learn a classification of drugs that enables them to immediately place a drug into a category that characterizes the likely pharmacology. In addition the main or original drug in each category (the prototype drug) should be thoroughly studied. The close relatives need merely to be known by name and with reference to their advantages over the prototype drug.

Though it may be obvious, it is still worth repeating that a minimum knowledge of prototype drugs consists of the following:

1. *Chemistry*. You should be able to recognize the structural formula. Are there any structure-activity relationships (SARs)? What is the main ring structure? steroid? quinoline? benzodiazepine? sympathetic amine? etc.

2. *Mechanism of Action*. This usually consists of two parts: (1) molecular and (2) cellular or physiologic. Mechanisms of action mainly explain pharmacodynamics or effects on organ systems that are of most use in a clinical knowledge of the drug. For example, does the drug lower blood pressure and, if so, does it do so by vasodilation, negative inotropic effects on the heart, central nervous sytem mechanisms, etc.?

3. *Pharmacokinetics*. This covers absorption, distribution, and elimination of the drug. What is the usual route of administration of the drug? What is its half-life, degree of protein binding, etc.? *The dose of the drug is usually not asked in modern examinations*. However, the means by which dosage can increase or decrease blood levels of drugs must be known. This is the essence of pharmacokinetics. Concepts and formulas for determining half-life, volume of distribution, and clearance must be understood and memorized. They are listed at the beginning of the first chapter, General Principles.

4. *Clinical Use*. You should know FDA indications plus medically accepted uses.

5. *Toxicity*. This includes adverse reactions and serious toxicities, such as nephritis, hepatitis, blood dyscrasia, etc. You should know important drug interactions.

With respect to names of drugs, the generic name must be known even though the trade name is often more commonly used. In this text, the generic name is always used and often, especially when it is a relatively new drug, the trade name is mentioned as well. It is advantageous to memorize certain endings because they give a clue as to the category in which a drug belongs; there are many exceptions, but these endings do help memory. The following are examples of endings of generic names:

Ending	Drug Class	Examples
-ane	volatile general anesthetics	halothane, enflurane
-azepam	antianxiety drugs	diazepam, lorazepam
-azine	phenothiazine-like antipsychotic drugs	chlorpromazine, thioridazine
-bital	barbiturate sedative hypnotic drugs	phenobarbital, secobarbital
-caine	local anesthetics	cocaine, procaine
-cillin	penicillins	nafcillin, piperacillin
-cycline	tetracycline-type antibiotics	doxycycline, methacycline
-mycin	aminoglycoside antibiotics	streptomycin, kanamycin
-olol	beta-adrenergic blockers	propranolol, metoprolol
-opril	angiotensin-converting enzyme inhibitors	captopril, enalapril
-statin	HMG-CoA reductase inhibitors	lovastatin, pravastatin
-zosin	postsynaptic alpha-receptor blockers	terazosin, prazosin

PRETEST®

Pharmacology

General Principles

Drug-Receptor Interaction
- Dose-response relationship
  - Graded dose-response curve
  - Quantal dose-response curve
  - Time-action curves
  - Therapeutic index
  - Drug assays, biologic vs chemical
- Receptors
  - Nature of the drug-receptor interaction
  - Structure and activity relationship (SAR)
  - Physical chemistry of the drug-receptor association
  - Relationship to Michaelis-Menten enzyme kinetics
- Simultaneous action of two drugs
  - Additive effects
  - Potentiation
  - Synergism
  - Competitive antagonism
  - Noncompetitive antagonism
- Other factors in drug-receptor interaction
  - Tolerance
  - Tachyphylaxis
  - Up and down regulation by the number of receptors
  - Scatchard plot

Molecular Models of Receptors and Transduction Mechanisms

1. Ion channel receptors
   - Nicotine
   - GABA
   - Glycine
   - Glutamate (NMDA, quisqualate, kainate)
   - Transduction mechanism = ionic
2. Receptor–G protein–effector system
   - Beta adrenergic
   - Muscarinic
   - Serotonin
   - Angiotensin
   - Rhodopsin
   - Transduction mechanism = G protein linked by guanine diphosphate and triphosphate (GDP-GTP) linked to adenylate-cyclase activity, phospholipase, potassium, and calcium channels
3. Receptor tyrosine kinases
   - Erythrocyte growth factor (EGF)
   - Platelet-derived growth factor (PDGF)
   - Insulin
   - Transduction mechanism = Activation of protein kinases
4. Steroid hormone receptors
   - Thyroid hormone
   - Vitamin D
   - Estrogen
   - Progesterone

- Glucocorticoid
  - Transduction mechanism = transcriptional changes by binding to DNA
- Biotransformation
  - Lipophilic versus hydrophilic considerations
  - Phase I reactions
    - Oxidations
    - Reductions
    - Hydrolysis
    - Effect on water solubility
  - Phase II reactions
    - Conjugations
      - Glucuronic acid
      - Glutathione
      - Sulfate
    - Effect on water solubility
  - Microsomal cytochrome P-450
    - Oxidation reactions
      - Aliphatic and aromatic hydroxylations
      - Epioxidation
      - N, O, and S dealkylation
      - Sulfoxidation
      - Desulfuration
      - Dehalogenation
  - Nonmicrosomal oxidations
    - Alcohol
    - Aldehyde
    - Monoamine
    - Diamine
    - Purine
  - Reduction reactions
    - Microsomal
      - Nitro, azo, dehalogenation
    - Nonmicrosomal
      - Aldehyde, ketone, quinine
  - Pharmacogenetic variants
    - Slow acetylators
    - Idiosyncratic reactions to drugs
- Pharmacokinetics
  - Types of absorption
    - Passive transport
    - Specialized transport
  - Sites of absorption
    - Alimentary canal
    - Oral mucosa
    - Rectal mucosa
    - Skin
  - Routes of administration
    - Parenteral
      - Intravenous
      - Intramuscular
      - Subcutaneous
    - Respiratory tract
      - Aerosols
    - Topical
  - Distribution
    - Lipid/water partition coefficient
    - Plasma protein binding
    - Tissue protein binding
  - Redistribution
  - Elimination
    - Renal excretion
    - Biotransformation
    - Biliary excretion
    - Minor in saliva, sweat, milk
  - Pharmacokinetic models and compartments
    - One compartment
    - Two compartments
  - Kinetics
    - First order
      - $\text{Slope} = \frac{-k}{2.303}$
      - Half-life ($t\frac{1}{2}$)
      - $t\frac{1}{2} = \frac{0.693}{k}$
  - Zero-order rate equation
  - Volume of distribution (V_d)
    - $V_d = \frac{\text{Total amount of drug in the body}}{\text{concentration of drug in plasma}}$
  - Distribution phase vs elimination

phase determined in plasma concentration × time curves

Clearance

$$CL_{total} = V_d \times k_e = \frac{0.693 \times V_d}{t^{1}\!/_{2}}$$

$$t^{1}\!/_{2} = \frac{0.693 \times V_d}{CL_{total}}$$

- Dosage regimens and pharmacokinetic profiles
  - Single doses
    - Intravenous
    - Oral
  - Bioavailability
  - Multiple doses
    - Interval between doses and accumulation
    - Continuous IV infusion
    - Multiple oral dosing

Clinical Pharmacology
- Definition and scope
- Statistical and epidemiologic approaches
- Bioavailability and bioequivalence
- Placebo effect

Drug Interactions
- Mechanisms
  - Enzyme stimulation (induction)
  - Enzyme inhibition
  - Gastrointestinal absorption changes
  - Protein binding
  - Adrenergic mechanisms
  - Cholinergic mechanisms
  - Neuromuscular junction
  - Drug biotransformation
  - Renal tubular transport
  - Urinary pH and drug excretion

Factors Affecting Drug Dosage
- Age, sex, and weight
- Pregnancy and lactation
- Renal disease
- Hepatic disease
- Pharmacogenetics

Development of New Drugs
- Animal vs human doses
- Single-dose methodology
- Open studies
- Blind and double-blind studies

Regulation by the Food and Drug Administration
- Investigational new drug (IND)
- New drug application (NDA)
- Phase I, II, III, and IV studies
- Postmarketing surveillance

Ethics of Human Investigation
- Institutional Review Board (IRB)

Fate of marketed drugs

DIRECTIONS: Each question below contains five suggested responses. Select the **one best** response to each question.

1. Of the many types of plots of data that are used to help explain the pharmacodynamics of drugs, which plot is very useful for determining the total number of receptors and the affinity of a drug for those receptors in a tissue or membrane?

(A) Graded dose-response curve
(B) Quantal dose-response curve
(C) Scatchard plot
(D) Double-reciprocal plot
(E) Michaelis-Menten plot

2. Which route of administration is most likely to subject a drug to a first-pass effect?

(A) Intravenous
(B) Inhalational
(C) Oral
(D) Sublingual
(E) Intramuscular

3. Two drugs may act on the same tissue or organ through independent receptors, resulting in effects in opposite directions. This is known as

(A) physiologic antagonism
(B) chemical antagonism
(C) competitive antagonism
(D) irreversible antagonism
(E) dispositional antagonism

Questions 4–7

A new aminoglycoside antibiotic (5 mg/kg) was infused intravenously over 30 min to a 70-kg volunteer. The plasma concentrations of the drug were measured at various times after the end of the infusion, as recorded in the table and shown in the figure below.

Time After Dosing Stopped (h)	Plasma Aminoglycoside Concentration (μg/mL)
0.0	18.0
0.5	10.0
1.0	5.8
2.0	4.6
3.0	3.7
4.0	3.0
5.0	2.4
6.0	1.9
8.0	1.3

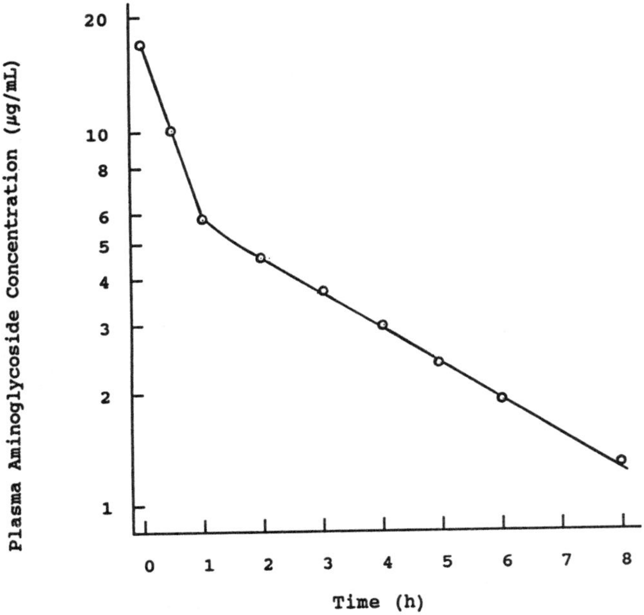

4. The elimination half-life ($t_{1/2}$) of the aminoglycoside in this patient was approximately

(A) 0.6 h
(B) 1.2 h
(C) 2.1 h
(D) 3.1 h
(E) 4.2 h

5. The elimination rate constant (k_e) of the aminoglycoside in this patient was approximately

(A) 0.15 h^{-1}
(B) 0.22 h^{-1}
(C) 0.33 h^{-1}
(D) 0.60 h^{-1}
(E) 1.13 h^{-1}

6. The apparent volume of distribution (V_d) of the drug in this patient was approximately

(A) 0.62 L
(B) 19 L
(C) 50 L
(D) 110 L
(E) 350 L

7. The total body clearance (CL_{total}) of the drug in this patient was approximately

(A) 11 L/h
(B) 23 L/h
(C) 35 L/h
(D) 47 L/h
(E) 65 L/h

8. If a drug is repeatedly administered at dosing intervals equal to its elimination half-life, the number of doses required for the plasma concentration of the drug to reach the steady state is

(A) 2 to 3
(B) 4 to 5
(C) 6 to 7
(D) 8 to 9
(E) 10 or more

9. The pharmacokinetic value that most reliably reflects the amount of drug reaching the target tissue after oral administration is the

(A) peak blood concentration
(B) time to peak blood concentration
(C) product of the volume of distribution and the first-order rate constant
(D) volume of distribution
(E) area under the blood concentration–time curve

10. It was determined that 95 percent of an oral 80-mg dose of verapamil (Calan, Isoptin) was absorbed in a 70-kg test subject. However, because of extensive biotransformation during its first pass through the portal circulation, the bioavailability of verapamil was only 25 percent. Assuming a liver blood flow of 1500 mL/min, the hepatic clearance of verapamil in this situation was

(A) 60 mL/min
(B) 375 mL/min
(C) 740 mL/min
(D) 1110 mL/min
(E) 1425 mL/min

11. Drug products have many types of names. Of the following types of names that are applied to drugs, the one that is the official name and refers only to that drug and not to a particular product is the

(A) generic name
(B) trade name
(C) brand name
(D) chemical name
(E) proprietary name

12. Which of the following is classified as belonging to the tyrosine kinase family of receptors?

(A) $GABA_A$ receptor
(B) β-Adrenergic receptor
(C) Insulin receptor
(D) Nicotinic-II receptor
(E) Hydrocortisone receptor

13. Identical doses of a capsule preparation (X) and a tablet preparation (Y) of the same drug were compared on a blood concentration–time plot with respect to peak concentration, time to peak concentration, and area under the curve after oral administration as shown in the figure below. This comparison was made to determine which of the following?

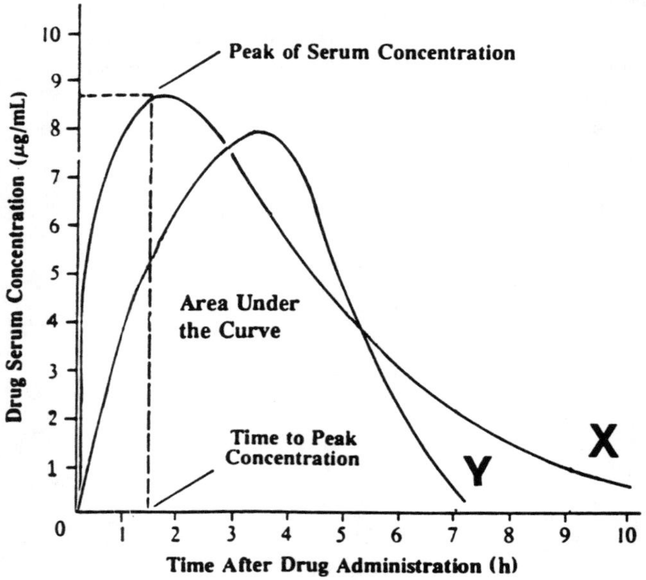

(A) Potency
(B) Extent of plasma protein binding
(C) Bioequivalence
(D) Therapeutic effectiveness
(E) None of the above

DIRECTIONS: Each numbered question or incomplete statement below is NEGATIVELY phrased. Select the **one best** lettered response.

14. All the following characteristics are associated with the process of facilitated diffusion of drugs EXCEPT

(A) the transport mechanism becomes saturated at high drug concentrations
(B) the process is selective for certain ionic or structural configurations of the drug
(C) if two compounds are transported by the same mechanism, one will competitively inhibit the transport of the other
(D) the drug crosses the membrane against a concentration gradient and the process requires cellular energy
(E) the transport process can be inhibited noncompetitively by substances that interfere with cellular metabolism

15. The route of excretion for drugs or their metabolic derivatives that is quantitatively the LEAST significant is which of the following?

(A) Biliary tract
(B) Kidneys
(C) Lungs
(D) Feces
(E) Milk

16. All the following are phase I biotransformation reactions EXCEPT

(A) sulfoxide formation
(B) nitro reduction
(C) ester hydrolysis
(D) sulfate conjugation
(E) deamination

17. An enteric-coated dosage form can be used to avoid all the following problems possible from oral drug administration EXCEPT

(A) irritation to the gastric mucosa with nausea and vomiting
(B) destruction of the drug by gastric acid or digestive enzymes
(C) unpleasant taste of the drug
(D) formation of nonabsorbable drug-food complexes
(E) variability in absorption caused by fluctuations in gastric emptying time

18. All the following statements concerning receptors bound to plasma membranes, their interaction with ligands, and the biologic response to this interaction are true EXCEPT

(A) structurally, these receptors have hydrophobic amino acid domains, which are in contact with the membrane, and hydrophilic regions, which extend into the extracellular fluid and the cytoplasm
(B) chemical interactions of ligands with these receptors may involve the formation of many types of bonds, including ionic, hydrogen, Van der Waals, and covalent
(C) ligand-receptor interactions are often stereospecific, i.e., one stereoisomer is usually more potent than the other
(D) a ligand that acts as an agonist at membrane-bound receptors increases the activity of an intracellular second messenger
(E) activation of membrane-bound receptors and subsequent intracellular events elicit a biologic response through the transcription of DNA

19. All the following statements concerning binding of drugs to plasma proteins are true EXCEPT

(A) acidic drugs generally bind to plasma albumin; basic drugs preferentially bind to α_1-acidic glycoprotein
(B) plasma protein binding is a reversible process
(C) binding sites on plasma proteins are nonselective and drugs with similar physicochemical characteristics compete for these limited sites
(D) the fraction of the drug in the plasma that is bound is inactive and generally unavailable for systemic distribution
(E) plasma protein binding generally limits renal tubular secretion and biotransformation

20. All the following compounds are prodrugs that are biotransformed to a pharmacologically active product EXCEPT

(A) minoxidil (Loniten)
(B) enalapril maleate (Vasotec)
(C) diazepam (Valium)
(D) sulfasalazine (Azulfidine)
(E) sulindac (Clinoril)

21. All the following statements concerning drug distribution into and out of the central nervous system (CNS) are true EXCEPT

(A) the blood-brain barrier, which involves drug movement through glial cell membranes as well as capillary membranes, is the main hindrance to drug distribution to the CNS
(B) most drugs enter the CNS by simple diffusion at rates proportional to the lipid solubility of the nonionized form of the drug
(C) receptor-mediated transport allows certain peptides to gain access to the brain
(D) strongly ionized drugs freely enter the CNS through carrier-mediated transport systems
(E) some drugs leave the CNS by passing from the cerebrospinal fluid into the dural blood sinuses through the arachnoid villi

22. The greater proportion of the dose of a drug administered orally will be absorbed in the small intestine. However, on the assumption that passive transport of the nonionized form of a drug determines its rate of absorption, which of the following compounds will be absorbed to the LEAST extent in the stomach?

(A) Ampicillin (pK_a = 2.5)
(B) Aspirin (pK_a = 3.0)
(C) Warfarin (pK_a = 5.0)
(D) Phenobarbital (pK_a = 7.4)
(E) Propranolol (pK_a = 9.4)

DIRECTIONS: Each group of questions below consists of lettered headings followed by a set of numbered items. For each numbered item select the **one** lettered heading with which it is **most** closely associated. Each lettered heading may be used **once, more than once, or not at all.**

Questions 23–25

For each type of drug interaction below, select the pair of substances that illustrates it with a *reduction* in drug effectiveness.

(A) Tetracycline and milk
(B) Amobarbital (Amytal) and secobarbital (Seconal)
(C) Isoproterenol (Isuprel) and propranolol (Inderal)
(D) Soap and benzalkonium chloride (Ionil)
(E) Sulfamethoxazole and trimethoprim

23. Therapeutic interaction

24. Physical interaction

25. Chemical interaction

Questions 26–28

For each description of a drug response below, choose the term with which it is most likely to be associated.

(A) Supersensitivity
(B) Tachyphylaxis
(C) Tolerance
(D) Hyposensitivity
(E) Anaphylaxis

26. Immunologically mediated reaction to drug observed soon after administration

27. A rapid reduction in the effect of a given dose of a drug after only one or two doses

28. Hyperreactivity to a drug seen as a result of denervation

Questions 29–33

Many families of drugs consist of members that vary only with respect to substituents on a common ring structure. For each pharmacologic effect listed, select the structure with which it is most likely to be associated.

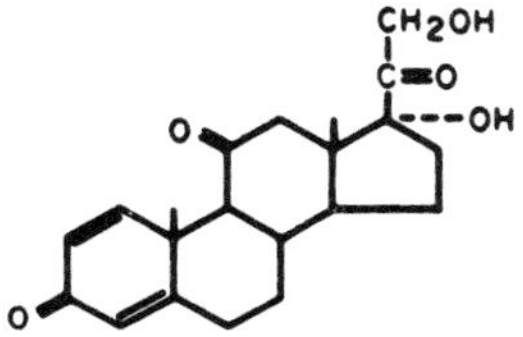

A

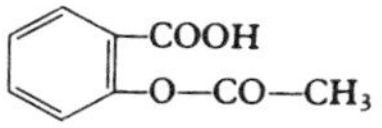

B

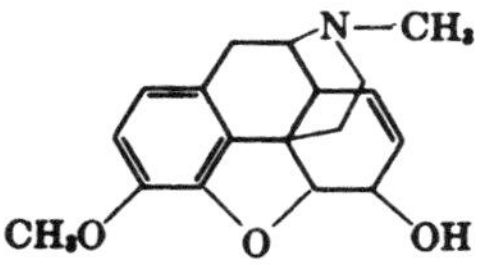

C

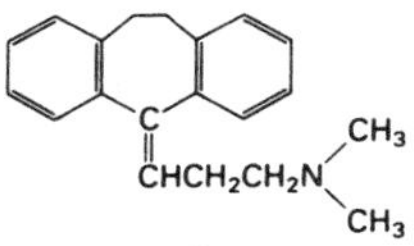

D

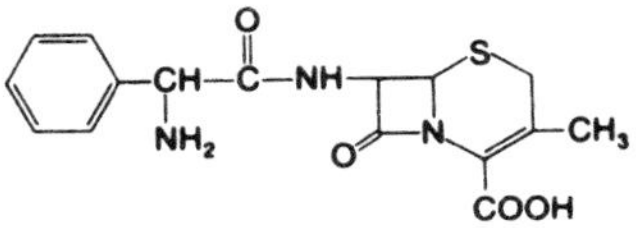

E

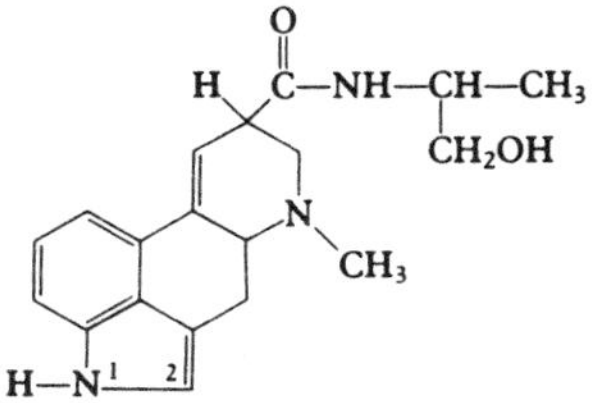

F

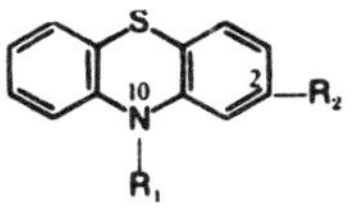

G

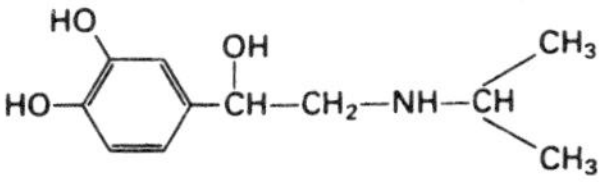

H

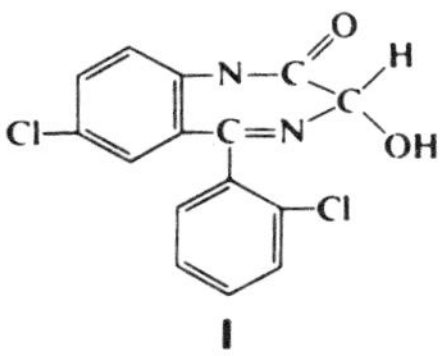

I

29. Bronchodilator

30. Opioid analgesic

31. Antipsychotic

32. Antimicrobial

33. Corticosteroid anti-inflammatory

Questions 34–36

For each component of a time-action curve listed below, choose the lettered interval (shown on the diagram) with which it is most closely associated.

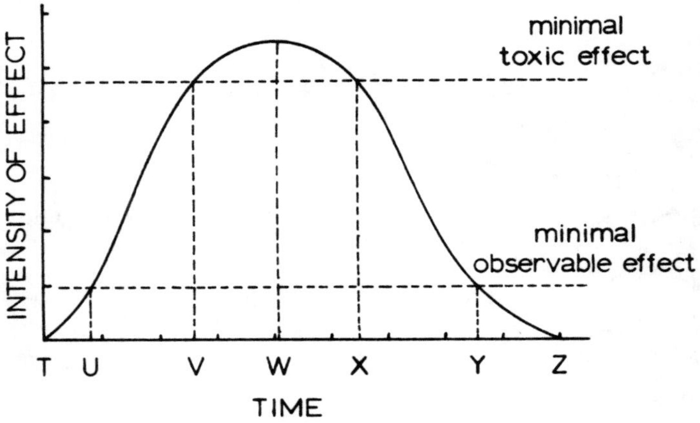

(A) T to U
(B) T to V
(C) T to W
(D) T to Z
(E) U to V
(F) U to W
(G) U to X
(H) U to Y
(I) V to X
(J) X to Y

34. Time to peak effect

35. Time to onset of action

36. Duration of action

Questions 37–39

For each description below, select the transmembranal transport mechanism it best defines.

(A) Filtration
(B) Simple diffusion
(C) Facilitated diffusion
(D) Active transport
(E) Endocytosis

37. Lipid-soluble drugs cross the membrane at a rate proportional to the concentration gradient across the membrane and the lipid: water partition coefficient of the drug

38. Bulk flow of water through membrane pores, resulting from osmotic differences across the membrane, transports drug molecules that fit through the membrane pores

39. After binding to a proteinaceous membrane carrier, drugs are carried across the membrane (with the expenditure of cellular energy), where they are released

Questions 40–42

Lipid-soluble xenobiotics are commonly biotransformed by oxidation in the drug-metabolizing microsomal system (DMMS). For each description below, choose the component of the microsomal mixed-function oxidase system with which it is most closely associated.

(A) NADPH
(B) Cytochrome *a*
(C) ATP
(D) NADPH–cytochrome P-450 reductase
(E) Monoamine oxidase
(F) Cyclooxygenase
(G) Cytochrome P-450

40. A group of iron-containing isoenzymes that activate molecular oxygen to a form capable of interacting with organic substrates

41. The component that provides reducing equivalents for the enzyme system

42. A flavoprotein that accepts reducing equivalents and transfers them to the catalytic enzyme

General Principles
Answers

1. The answer is C. *(DiPalma, 4/e, pp 22–23. Gilman, 8/e, pp 44–45.)* Based upon the concept that, for most situations, the association of a drug with its receptor is reversible, the following reaction applies:

$$D + R \underset{k_2}{\overset{k_1}{\rightleftarrows}} DR \rightarrow \text{Effect}$$

where D is the concentration of free drug, R is the concentration of receptors, DR is the concentration of drug bound to its receptors, and K_D (equal to k_2/k_1) is the equilibrium dissociation constant. The affinity of a drug for its receptor is estimated from the dissociation constant in that its reciprocal, $1/K_D$, is the affinity constant. All the plots listed in the question can be used to quantitate some aspect of drug action. For example, K_D can be determined from the Michaelis-Menten relationship, graded dose-response curves, and the Scatchard plot. However, only the Scatchard plot can be used to determine the total number of receptors in a tissue or membrane. This is accomplished by measuring the binding of a radioactively labeled drug to a membrane or tissue preparation in vitro. A Scatchard plot of the binding of ^{3}H-yohimbine to α_2-adrenergic receptors on human platelet membranes is shown on the facing page as an example. A plot of DR/D (bound/free drug) versus DR (bound drug) yields a slope of $1/K_D$ (the affinity constant) and an x intercept of R (total number of receptors).

This type of analysis is very useful in certain therapeutic situations. For example, Scatchard analysis is used to determine the number of estrogen receptors present in a biopsy of breast tissue prior to developing a drug treatment regimen for breast cancer in a patient.

2. The answer is C. *(DiPalma, 4/e, pp 48–49, 61–62. Gilman, 8/e, p 5.)* The first-pass effect is commonly considered to involve the biotransformation of a drug during its first passage through the portal circulation of the liver. Drugs that are administered orally and rectally enter the portal circulation of the liver and can be biotransformed by this organ prior to reaching the systemic circulation. Therefore, drugs with a *high* first-pass effect are highly biotransformed quickly, which reduces the oral bioavailability and the systemic blood concentrations of the compounds. Administration by the intravenous, in-

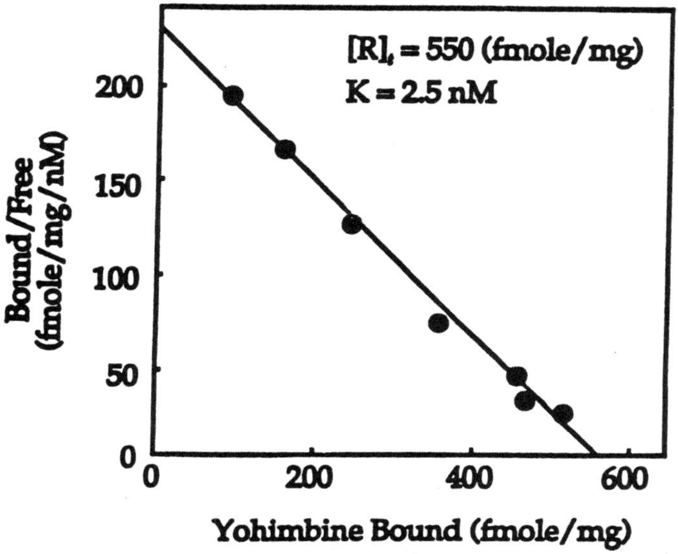

(From Neubig RR, Gantros RD, and Brasier RS: *Mol Pharmacol* 28:475–486, 1985, with permission.)

tramuscular, and sublingual routes allows the drug to attain concentrations in the systemic circulation and to be distributed throughout the body prior to hepatic metabolism. In most cases, drugs administered by inhalation are not subjected to a significant first-pass effect unless the respiratory tissue is a major site for the drug's biotransformation.

3. The answer is A. *(DiPalma, 4/e, p 24. Gilman, 8/e, pp 53–54.) Physiologic,* or *functional, antagonism* occurs when two drugs produce opposite effects on the same physiologic function, often by interacting with different types of receptors. A practical example of this is the use of epinephrine as a bronchodilator to counteract the bronchoconstriction that occurs following histamine release from mast cells in the respiratory tract during a severe allergic reaction. Histamine constricts the bronchioles by stimulating histamine H_1 receptors in the tissue; epinephrine relaxes this tissue through its agonistic activity on β_2-adrenergic receptors.

Chemical antagonism results when two drugs combine with each other chemically and the activity of one or both is blocked. For example, dimercaprol chelates lead and reduces the toxicity of this heavy metal. *Competitive antagonism*, or *inactivation*, occurs when two compounds compete for the same receptor site; this is a reversible interaction. Thus, atropine blocks the effects of acetylcholine on the heart by competing with the neurotransmitter for binding to cardiac muscarinic receptors. *Irreversible antagonism* generally results from the binding of an antagonist to the same receptor site as the agonist by covalent interaction or by a very slowly dissociating non-covalent interaction. An example of this antagonism is the blockade produced by phenoxybenzamine on α-adrenergic receptors, resulting in a long-lasting reduction in the activity of norepinephrine. *Dispositional antagonism* occurs when one drug alters the pharmacokinetics (absorption, distribution, biotransformation, or excretion) of a second drug so that less of the active compound reaches the target tissue. For example, phenobarbital induces the biotransformation of warfarin, reducing its anticoagulant activity.

4. The answer is D. *(DiPalma, 4/e, pp 55–58. Katzung, 6/e, p 40.)* The figure shows an elimination pattern with two distinct components, which typifies a two-compartment model. The upper portion of the line represents the α phase, which is the distribution of the drug from the tissues that receive high rates of blood flow (the central compartment, e.g., the brain, heart, kidney, and lungs) to the tissues with lower rates of blood flow (the peripheral compartment, e.g., skeletal muscle, adipose tissue, and bone). Once distribution to all tissue is complete, equilibrium occurs throughout the body. The elimination of the drug from the body (the β phase) is represented by the lower linear portion of the line; this part of the line is used to determine the elimination half-life of the drug.

At 2 h after dosing, the plasma concentration was 4.6 μg/mL; at 5 h the concentration was 2.4 μg/mL. Therefore the plasma concentration of this aminoglycoside decreased to one-half in approximately 3 h—its half-life. In addition, drug elimination usually occurs according to first-order kinetics, i.e., a linear relationship is obtained when the drug concentration is plotted on a logarithmic scale versus time on an arithmetic scale (a semilogarithmic plot).

5. The answer is B. *(DiPalma, 4/e, pp 57–58. Katzung, 6/e, p 39.)* The fraction change in drug concentration per unit of time for any first-order process is expressed by the elimination rate constant, k_e. This constant is related to the half-life ($t_{1/2}$) by the equation $k_e t_{1/2} = 0.693$. The units of the elimination rate constant are time^{-1}, while the $t_{1/2}$ is expressed in units of time. By substitution of the appropriate value for half-life estimated from the data from the graph or table (the β phase) into the above equation, rearranged to solve for k_e, the answer is calculated as follows:

$$k_e = \frac{0.693}{t_{1/2}} = \frac{0.693}{3.0\ \text{h}} = 0.23\ \text{h}^{-1}$$

The problem can also be solved mathematically:

$$\log[A] = \log[A_o] - \frac{k_e}{2.303}\,t$$

where $[A_o]$ is the initial drug concentration, [A] is the final drug concentration, t is the time interval between the two values, and k_e is the elimination rate constant. For example, by solving for k_e using the plasma concentration values at 2 and 5 h,

$$\log[2.4\ \mu g/mL] = \log[4.6\ \mu g/mL] - \frac{k_e}{2.303}\,3h$$

k_e will equal 0.22 h^{-1}.

6. **The answer is C.** *(DiPalma, 4/e, pp 58–60. Katzung, 6/e, p 38.)* The apparent volume of distribution is defined as the volume of fluid into which a drug appears to distribute with a concentration equal to that of plasma, or the volume of fluid necessary to dissolve the drug and yield the same concentration as that found in plasma. By convention, the value of the plasma concentration at zero time is used. In this problem, a hypothetical plasma concentration of the drug at zero time (7 μg/mL) can be estimated by extrapolating the linear portion of the elimination curve (the β phase) back to zero time. Therefore, the apparent volume of distribution (V_d) is calculated by

$$V_d = \frac{\text{Total amount of drug in the body}}{\text{Drug concentration in plasma at zero time}}$$

Since the total amount of drug in the body is the intravenous dose, 350 mg, i.e., 5 mg/kg × 70 kg, and the estimated plasma concentration at zero time is 7μg/mL, substitution of these numbers in the equation yields the apparent volume of distribution:

$$V_d = \frac{350\text{ mg}}{7\ \mu g/mL} = 50\text{ L}$$

7. **The answer is A.** *(DiPalma, 4/e, p 60. Katzung, 6/e, pp 39–40.)* Clearance by an organ is defined as the apparent volume of a biologic fluid from which a drug is removed by elimination processes per unit of time. The total body clearance (CL_{total}) is defined as the sum of clearances of all the organs and tissues that eliminate a drug. CL_{total} is influenced by the apparent volume of distribution (V_d) and the elimination rate constant (k_e). The more rapidly a drug is cleared, the greater is the value of CL_{total}. Therefore, for the new aminoglycoside in this patient,

$$CL_{total} = V_d k_e = (50\ \text{L})\ (0.22\ \text{h}^{-1}) = 11\ \text{L/h}$$

8. The answer is B. *(DiPalma, 4/e, pp 62–63. Gilman, 8/e, pp 26–27.)* When a drug is administered in multiple doses and each dose is given prior to the complete elimination of the previous dose, the mean plasma concentration (C) of the drug during each dose interval rises as shown in the following figure:

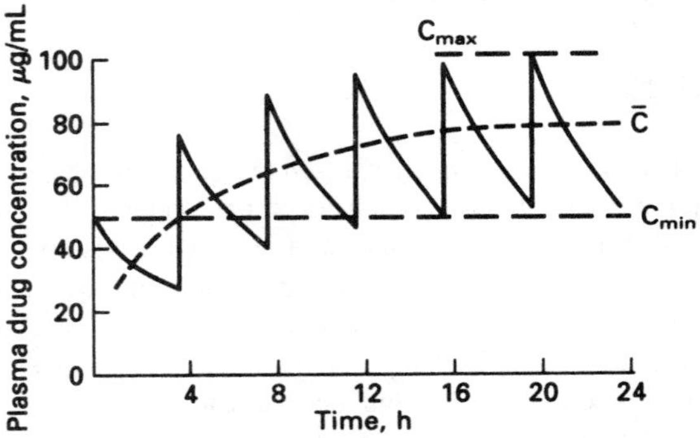

(From DiPalma and DiGregorio, with permission.)

The plasma concentration will continue to rise until it reaches a plateau, or steady state. At this time, the plasma concentration will fluctuate between a maximum (C_{max}) and a minimum (C_{min}) level, but, more importantly, the amount of drug eliminated per dose interval will equal the amount of drug absorbed per dose. When a drug is given at a dosing interval equal to its elimination half-life, it will reach 50 percent of its steady state plasma concentration after one half-life, 75 percent after two half-lives, 87.5 percent after three, 93.75 percent after four, and 96.87 percent after five. Thus, from a practical viewpoint, regardless of the magnitude of the dose or the half-life, the steady state will be achieved in four to five half-lives.

9. The answer is E. *(DiPalma, 4/e, pp 61–62. Gilman, 8/e, p 25.)* The fraction of a drug dose absorbed after oral administration is affected by a wide variety of factors that can strongly influence the peak blood levels and the time to peak blood concentration. The volume of distribution and the total body clearance (volume of distribution × first-order elimination rate constant) also are important in determining the amount of drug that reaches the target tissue. Only the area under the blood concentration–time curve, however, reflects absorption, distribution, metabolism, and excretion factors; it is the most reliable and popular method of evaluating bioavailability.

10. The answer is D. *(DiPalma, 4/e, pp 48, 60–62, 77. Gilman, 8/e, pp 5, 21.)* Bioavailability is defined as the fraction or percentage of a drug that becomes available to the systemic circulation following administration by any route. This takes into consideration that not all of an orally administered drug is absorbed and that a drug can be removed from the plasma and biotransformed by the liver during its initial passage through the portal circulation. A bioavailability of 25 percent indicates that only 20 mg of the 80-mg dose (i.e., 80 mg × 0.25 = 20 mg) reached the systemic circulation. Organ clearance can be determined by knowing the blood flow through the organ (Q) and the extraction ratio (ER) for the drug by the organ, according to the equation

$$CL_{organ} = (Q) \times (ER)$$

The extraction ratio is dependent upon the amounts of drug entering (C_i) and exiting (C_o) the organ; i.e.,

$$ER = \frac{(C_i) - (C_o)}{(C_i)}$$

In this problem the amount of verapamil entering the liver was 76 mg (80 mg × 0.95) and the amount leaving was 20 mg. Therefore,

$$ER = \frac{76 \text{ mg} - 20 \text{ mg}}{76 \text{ mg}} = 0.74$$

$$CL_{liver} = (1500 \text{ mL/min})\ (0.74) = 1110 \text{ mL/min}$$

11. The answer is A. *(AMA Drug Evaluations Annual 1994, pp 4, 10–11, 14–15.)* When a new chemical entity is first synthesized by a pharmaceutical company, it is given a *chemical name*, e.g., acetylsalicylic acid. During the process of investigation of the usefulness of the new chemical as a drug, it is given a *generic name* by the United States Adopted Names (USAN) Council, which negotiates with the pharmaceutical manufacturer in the choice of a meaningful and distinctive generic name for the new drug. This name will be the established, official name that can only be applied to that one unique drug compound, e.g., aspirin. The *trade name* (or *brand name*, or *proprietary name*) is a registered name given to the product by the pharmaceutical company that is manufacturing or distributing the drug and identifies a particular product containing that drug, e.g., Ecotrin. Thus, *acetylsalicylic acid, aspirin,* and

Ecotrin, for example, all refer to the same therapeutic drug entity; however, only *aspirin* is the official generic name.

12. The answer is C. *(DiPalma, 4/e, pp 29–40. Gilman, 8/e, pp 35–38.)* There are four major classes of receptors: (1) ion channel receptors, (2) receptors coupled to G proteins, (3) receptors with tyrosine-specific kinase activity, and (4) receptors for steroid hormones. In most cases, drugs that act via receptors do so by binding to extracellular receptors that transduce the information intracellularly by a variety of mechanisms. Activated ion channel receptors enhance the influx of extracellular ions into the cell; for example, the nicotinic-II cholinergic receptor selectively opens a channel for sodium ions and the $GABA_A$ receptor functions as an ionophore for chloride ions. Receptors coupled to G proteins (i.e., guanine nucleotide–binding proteins) act either by opening an ion channel or by stimulating or inhibiting specific enzymes (e.g., β-adrenergic receptor stimulation leads to an increase in cellular adenylate cyclase activity). When stimulated, receptors with tyrosine-specific protein kinase activity activate this enzyme to enhance the transport of ions and nutrients across the cell membrane; for example, insulin receptors function in this manner and increase glucose transport into insulin-dependent tissues. Steroid hormone receptors are different from all the above in that they are associated with the nucleus of the cell and are activated by steroid hormones (e.g., hydrocortisone) that penetrate into target cells. These receptors interact with DNA to enhance genetic transcription.

13. The answer is C. *(DiPalma, 4/e, pp 77–78. Katzung, 6/e, p 41.)* Drug absorption can vary significantly depending upon the product formulation used and the route of administration. The degree to which a drug achieves a particular concentration in the blood following administration by a route other than intravenous injection is a measure of its efficiency of absorption—its *bioavailability*. When a drug is produced by different processes (e.g., at different manufacturing sites or using different manufacturing or production techniques) or in a different dosage form (e.g., capsule, tablet, suspension) and contains the same amount of active ingredient and is to be used for the same therapeutic purpose, the extent to which the bioavailability of one dosage form differs from that of another must be evaluated. In the body, these dosage forms should produce similar blood, plasma, or blood concentration–time curves. The comparison of the bioavailability of two such dosage forms is called *bioequivalence*.

The bioequivalence of different preparations is assessed by an evaluation of three parameters: (1) the peak height concentration achieved by the drug in the dosage form, (2) the time to reach the peak concentration of the drug, and (3) the area under the concentration-time curve. The ascending limb of the curve is considered to be a general reflection of the rate of drug absorption from the dosage form. The descending limb of the concentration-time curve is a general indication of the rate of elimination of the drug from the body.

None of the other choices in the question (i.e., potency, effectiveness, or plasma protein binding) can be evaluated using this type of comparison.

14. The answer is D. *(DiPalma, 4/e, pp 45–46. Gilman, 8/e, pp 4–5.)* Drugs can be transferred across biologic membranes by passive processes (i.e., filtration and simple diffusion) and by specialized processes (i.e., active transport, facilitated diffusion, and pinocytosis). Active transport is a carrier-mediated process that shows all the characteristics listed in the question. Facilitated diffusion is similar to active transport except that the drug is *not* transported against a concentration gradient and *no* energy is required for this carrier-mediated system to function. Pinocytosis usually involves transport of proteins and macromolecules by a complex process in which a cell engulfs the compound within a membrane-bound vesicle.

15. The answer is E. *(DiPalma, 4/e, pp 52–54. Gilman, 8/e, pp 18–20.)* The amounts of drugs excreted in milk are small compared with those excreted by other routes; but drugs in milk may have significant, undesired pharmacologic effects on breast-fed infants. The principal route of excretion of the products of a given drug varies with the drug. Some drugs are predominantly excreted by the kidneys, whereas others leave the body in the bile and feces. Inhalation anesthetic agents are eliminated by the lungs. The path of excretion may affect the clinical choice of a drug, as is the case with renal failure or hepatic insufficiency.

16. The answer is D. *(DiPalma, 4/e, pp 65–72. Gilman, 8/e, pp 13–17.)* Biotransformation reactions involving the oxidation, reduction, or hydrolysis of a drug are classified as phase I (or nonsynthetic) reactions; these chemical reactions may result in either the activation or inactivation of a pharmacologic agent. There are many types of these reactions; oxidations are the most numerous. Phase II (or synthetic) reactions, which almost always result in the formation of an inactive product, involve conjugation of the drug (or its derivative) with an amino acid, carbohydrate, acetate, or sulfate. The conjugated form(s) of the drug or its derivatives may be more easily excreted than the parent compound.

17. The answer is E. *(DiPalma, 4/e, p 47.)* Tasteless enteric-coated tablets and capsules are formulated to resist the acidic pH found in the stomach. Once the preparation has passed into the intestine, the coating dissolves in the alkaline milieu and releases the drug. Therefore, gastric irritation, drug destruction by gastric acid, and the forming of complexes of the drug with food constituents will be avoided.

18. The answer is E. *(DiPalma, 4/e, pp 20–21, 28–30. Gilman, 8/e, pp 34–38.)* Based upon the molecular mechanisms with which receptors transduce signals, four major classes of receptors have been identified: (1) ion channel receptors, (2) receptors that interact with guanine nucleotide–binding proteins (G proteins), (3) receptors with tyrosine kinase activity, and (4) nuclear receptors. The first three types of receptors are complex membrane-bound proteins with hydrophilic regions located within the lipoid cell membrane and hydrophilic portions found protruding into the cytoplasm of the cell and the extracellular milieu; when activated, all of these receptors transmit (or transduce) information presented at the extracellular surface into ionic or biochemical signals within the cell, i.e., second messengers.

Nuclear receptors are found in the nucleus of the cell, not bound to plasma membranes. In addition, these receptors do not transduce information by second messenger systems; rather, they bind to nuclear chromatin and elicit a biologic response through the transcription of DNA and alterations in the formation of cellular proteins.

Ligand binding to all types of receptors may involve the formation of ionic, hydrogen, hydrophobic, Van der Waals, and covalent bonds. In most cases, ligand-receptor interactions are stereospecific; for example, natural (−)-epinephrine is 1000 times more potent than (+)-epinephrine.

19. The answer is E. *(DiPalma, 4/e, pp 51–52. Gilman, 8/e, pp 11–12.)* Since only the free (unbound) fraction of drug can cross biologic membranes, binding to plasma proteins limits a drug's concentration in tissues and therefore decreases the apparent volume of distribution of the drug. Plasma protein binding will also reduce glomerular filtration of the drug since this process is highly dependent on the free drug fraction. Renal tubular secretion and biotransformation of drugs are generally not limited by plasma protein binding because these processes reduce the free drug concentration in the plasma. If a drug is avidly transported through the tubule by the secretion process or rapidly biotransformed, the rates of these processes may exceed the rate of dissociation of the drug-protein complex (in order to restore the free: bound drug ratio in plasma) and thus becomes the rate-limiting factor for drug elimination. This assumes that equilibrium conditions exist and other influences, e.g., changes in pH or the presence of other drugs, do not occur.

20. The answer is C. *(DiPalma, 4/e, pp 52, 66. Gilman, 8/e, pp 13, 352–354, 425–426, 650, 661, 760, 801.)* Prodrugs are pharmacologically inactive compounds that, after administration, are converted to an active drug.

All the drugs listed are biotransformed to active products; however, only diazepam itself is active and, therefore, is not a prodrug. Diazepam, an active anxiolytic, can be converted to at least three active products: desmethyldiazepam (nordazepam), 3-hydroxydiazepam, and oxazepam (Serax), the last marketed as an antianxiety drug. Minoxidil is oxidized to minoxidil N-O sulfate, the active vasodilator antihypertensive; enalapril is hydrolyzed to form enalaprilat, a potent angiotensin converting enzyme inhibitor; sulfasalazine is cleaved to release its active component mesalamine, an anti-inflammatory agent used for its local action on the bowel; and sulindac is reduced to sulindac sulfide, a nonsteroidal anti-inflammatory drug.

21. The answer is D. *(DiPalma, 4/e, pp 50–51. Gilman, 8/e, p 11.)* Drugs can enter the brain from the circulation by passing through the blood-brain barrier. This boundary consists of several membranes including those of the capillary wall, the glial cells closely surrounding the capillary, and the neuron. In most cases, lipid-soluble drugs diffuse through these membranes at rates related to their lipid-to-water partition coefficients. Therefore, the greater the lipid solubility of the nonionized fraction of a weak acid or base, the more freely permeable the drug is to the brain. Some drugs enter the central nervous system (CNS) through specific carrier-mediated or receptor-mediated transport processes. Carrier-mediated systems appear to be involved predominantly in the transport of a variety of nutrients through the blood-brain barrier; however, the thyroid hormone triiodothyronine and drugs such as levodopa and methyldopa, which are structural derivatives of phenylalanine, cross the blood-brain barrier via carrier-mediated transport. Receptor-mediated transport functions to permit peptide, e.g., insulin, to enter the CNS; therefore, some peptide-like drugs are believed to gain access to the brain by this mechanism. Regardless of the process by which drugs can enter the CNS, strongly ionized drugs, e.g., quaternary amines, are unable to enter the CNS from the blood.

The exit of drugs from the CNS can involve (1) diffusion across the blood-brain barrier in the reverse direction at rates determined by the lipid solubility and degree of ionization of the drug, (2) drainage from the cerebrospinal fluid (CSF) into the dural blood sinuses by flowing through the wide channels of the arachnoid villi, and (3) active transport of certain organic anions and cations from the CSF to blood across the choroid plexuses.

22. The answer is E. *(Gilman, 8/e, pp 4–5. Katzung, 6/e, pp 2–3.)* Weak acids and weak bases are dissociated into nonionized and ionized forms depending upon the pK_a of the molecule and the pH of the environment. The nonionized form of a drug passes through cellular membranes more easily than the ionized form because it is more lipid-soluble. Thus, the rate of passive transport varies with the proportion of the drug that is nonionized. When the pH of the environment in which a weak acid or weak base drug is contained is equal to the pK_a, the drug is 50 percent dissociated. Weak acids (e.g., salicylates, barbiturates) are more readily absorbed from the stomach than from other regions of the alimentary canal because a large percentage of these weak acids are in the nonionized state. The magnitude of this effect can be estimated by applying the Henderson-Hasselbalch equation:

$$\log \left(\frac{\text{Protonated form}}{\text{Unprotonated form}}\right) = \text{p}K_a - \text{pH}$$

At an acidic pH of about 3, of the drugs in question all are weak acids except propranolol; therefore, propranolol has the greatest percentage of its molecules in the ionized form in the stomach. The higher the value of the pK_a, the less ionized these substances are in the stomach.

23–25. The answers are 23-C, 24-D, 25-A. *(DiPalma, 4/e, pp 81–82. Gilman, 8/e, pp 229, 358, 1054, 1119. Katzung, 6/e, pp 12–13, 17–18.)* A therapeutic drug interaction that reduces drug effectiveness results when two drugs with opposing pharmacologic effects are administered. For example, isoproterenol, a β-adrenergic stimulator, will antagonize the effect of propranolol, a β-adrenergic blocking agent. The combined use of amobarbital and secobarbital, both barbiturate sedative-hypnotics, represents a drug interaction that causes an *additive* (enhanced) pharmacologic response, i.e., depression of the central nervous system. The combination of the antimicrobials sulfamethoxazole and trimethoprim (Bactrim, Septra) is an example of a very useful drug interaction in which one drug *potentiates* the effects of another.

Physical interactions result when precipitation or another change in the physical state or solubility of a drug occurs. A common physical drug interaction takes place in the mixture of oppositely charged organic molecules, e.g., cationic (benzalkonium chloride) and anionic (soap) detergents.

Chemical drug interactions result when two administered substances combine with each other chemically. Tetracyclines complex with calcium (in milk), with aluminum and magnesium (often components of antacids), and with iron (in some multiple vitamins) to reduce the absorption of the tetracycline antibiotic.

26–28. The answers are 26-E, 27-B, 28-A. *(DiPalma, 4/e, pp 126, 375. Katzung, 6/e, pp 23, 813–814.)* Anaphylaxis refers to an acute hypersensitivity reaction that appears to be mediated primarily by IgE. Specific antigens can interact with these antibodies and cause sensitized mast cells to release vasoactive substances, such as histamine. Anaphylaxis to penicillin is one of the best known examples; the drug of choice to relieve the symptoms is epinephrine.

Decreased sensitivity to a drug, or tolerance, is seen with some drugs such as opiates and usually requires repeated administration of the drug. Tachyphylaxis, in contrast, is tolerance that develops rapidly, often after a single injection of drug. In some cases this may be due to what is termed the *down regulation* of drug receptors, in which the number of receptors becomes decreased.

A person who responds to an unusually low dose of a drug is called *hyperreactive*. Supersensitivity refers to increased responses to low doses only after denervation of an organ. At least three mechanisms are responsible for supersensitivity: increased receptors, reduction in tonic neuronal activity, and decreased neurotransmitter uptake mechanisms.

29–33. The answers are 29-H, 30-C, 31-G, 32-E, 33-A. *(DiPalma, 4/e, pp 117, 202, 245, 276, 290, 333, 346, 642.)* The steroid nucleus, exemplified by prednisone, is shown in Figure A. This is the structural basis for androgens, estrogens, progestogens, and anti-inflammatory corticosteroids.

Figure B is aspirin, a compound that can be categorized as a nonsteroidal anti-inflammatory drug, a nonopioid analgesic, and an antipyretic. Chemically, aspirin belongs to a group of compounds known as salicylates, which includes drugs such as salicylic acid, methylsalicylate, and salsalate.

Figure C illustrates codeine, a derivative of morphine, which contains the pentacyclic opioid structure. Although principally important for their analgesic activity, many opioids are also useful as antidiarrheals, respiratory depressants, and cough suppressants.

Amitriptyline is shown in Figure D. This compound is a member of a large group of compounds known as *tricyclic antidepressants*. The three-ring structure is similar to that of the phenothiazines (Figure G), but the pharmacologic properties are quite different. Other drugs included in this group are imipramine, desipramine, trimipramine, doxepin, and nortriptyline.

Figure E is the compound cephalexin, an important antimicrobial in the treatment of systemic bacterial infections. The four-membered β-lactam ring found in all the cephalosporin antibiotics is also contained within the structure of the penicillin derivatives.

Figure F represents a group of compounds known as *lysergic acid derivatives*, or *ergot alkaloids*, since all are derived from ergot, which is a product of a fungal infestation of grains, particularly rye. The compound shown is ergotamine, a useful vasoconstrictor and a drug used for relieving migraine headaches. Other ergot derivatives include ergonovine (an oxytocic) and bromocriptine (a drug used in the treatment of Parkinson's disease and hyperprolactinemia). These compounds are also structurally related to lysergic acid diethylamide (LSD).

Figure G is the phenothiazine nucleus, attachments to the nitrogen atom of which account principally for the differences in the pharmacokinetics of the various compounds that comprise this group. Examples include the piperazines, such as trifluoperazine; the piperidines, such as thioridazine; and the propylamines, or open-chain compounds, such as chlorpromazine. All of these agents are effective antipsychotic drugs.

Figure H is isoproterenol, a representative of a large class of sympathomimetic compounds, many of which are catecholamine derivatives that stimulate β-adrenergic receptors in bronchiolar smooth muscle, thus inducing the bronchioles to relax. Isoproterenol and structurally similar compounds (epinephrine, albuterol, terbutaline, metaproterenol, and isoetharine) are important bronchodilators used in the therapy of chronic obstructive pulmonary diseases, such as bronchial asthma.

Lorazepam is shown in Figure I. This antianxiety drug is representative of the benzodiazepines, compounds with antianxiety, anticonvulsant, skeletal muscle relaxant, and sedative properties.

Although it is not necessary to know the exact structure of each drug, knowledge of the basic structural characteristics of each class of drugs helps to categorize information and to predict the general properties and effects of some new compounds as they occur.

34–36. The answers are 34-C, 35-A, 36-H. *(DiPalma, 4/e, pp 19–20.)* Time-action curves relate the changes in intensity of the action of a drug dose and the times that these changes occur. There are three distinct phases that characterize the time-action pattern of most drugs: (1) The *time to onset of action* is from the moment of administration (T on the figure) to the time when the first drug effect is detected (U). (2) The *time to reach the peak effect* is from administration (T) until the maximum effect has occurred (W), regardless of whether this is above or below the level that produces some toxic effect. (3) The *duration of action* is described as the time from the appearance of a drug effect (U) until the effect disappears (Y). For some drugs a fourth phase occurs (interval Y to Z), in which *residual effects* of the drug may be present. These are usually undetectable, but may be uncovered by readministration of the same drug dose (observed as an increase in potency) or by administration of another drug (leading to some drug-drug interaction).

37–39. The answers are 37-B, 38-A, 39-D. *(DiPalma, 4/e, pp 45–46.)* The absorption, distribution, and elimination of drugs require that they cross various cellular membranes. The descriptions given in the question define the various transport mechanisms. The most common method by which ionic compounds of low molecular weight (100 to 200) enter cells is via membrane channels. The degree to which such filtration occurs varies from cell type to cell type because their pore sizes differ.

Simple diffusion is another mechanism by which substances cross membranes without the active participation of components in the membranes. Generally, lipid-soluble substances employ this method to enter cells. Both simple diffusion and filtration are dominant factors in most drug absorption, distribution, and elimination.

Pinocytosis is a type of endocytosis that is responsible for the transport of large molecules such as proteins and colloids. Some cell types—for example, endothelial cells—employ this transport mechanism extensively, but its importance in drug action is uncertain.

Membrane carriers are proteinaceous components of the cell membrane that are capable of combining with a drug at one surface of the membrane. The carrier-solute complex moves across the membrane, the solute is released, and the carrier then returns to the original surface where it can combine with another molecule of solute. There are two primary types of carrier-mediated transport: *active transport* and *facilitated diffusion.* During active transport (1) the drug crosses the membrane against a concentration gradient, (2) the transport mechanism becomes saturated at high drug concentrations and thus shows a *transport maximum*, and (3) the process is selective for certain structural configurations of the drug. Active transport is responsible for the movement of a number of organic acids and bases across membranes of renal tubules, choroid plexuses, and hepatic cells. With facilitated diffusion, the transport process is selective and saturable, but the drug is *not* transferred against a concentration gradient and does *not* require the expenditure of cellular energy. Glucose transport into erythrocytes is a good example of this process. In both situations, if two compounds are transported by the same mechanism, one will competitively inhibit the transport of the other and the transport process can be inhibited noncompetitively by substances that interfere with cellular metabolism.

40–42. The answers are 40-G, 41-A, 42-D. *(DiPalma, 4/e, pp 66–69. Katzung, 6/e, pp 51–54.)* There are four major components to the mixed-function oxidase system: (1) cytochrome P-450, (2) NADPH, or reduced nicotinamide adenine dinucleotide phosphate, (3) NADPH–cytochrome P-450 reductase, and (4) molecular oxygen. The figure shows the catalytic cycle for the reactions dependent upon cytochrome P-450.

Cytochrome P-450 catalyzes a diverse number of oxidative reactions involved in drug biotransformation; it undergoes reduction and oxidation during its catalytic cycle. A prosthetic group composed of iron and protoporphyrin IX (forming heme) binds molecular oxygen and converts it to an "activated" form for interaction with the drug substrate. Similar to hemoglobin, cytochrome P-450 is inhibited by carbon monoxide. This interaction results in an absorbance spectrum peak at 450 nm, hence the name *P-450.*

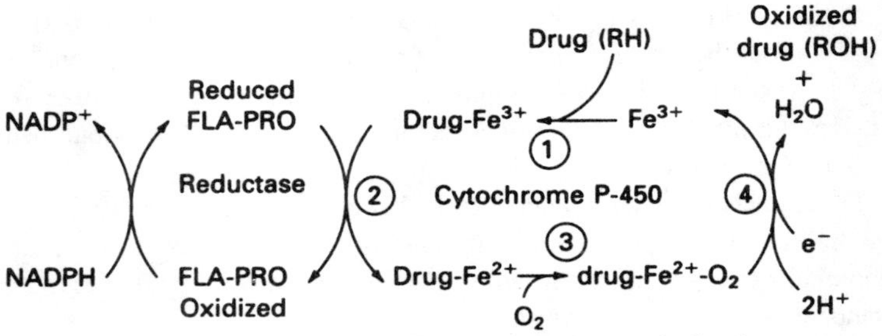

(From DiPalma and DiGregorio, with permission.)

NADPH gives up hydrogen atoms to the flavoprotein NADPH–cytochrome P-450 reductase and becomes $NADP^+$. The reduced flavoprotein transfers these reducing equivalents to cytochrome P-450. The reducing equivalents are used to activate molecular oxygen for incorporation into the substrate, as described above. Thus NADPH provides the reducing equivalents, while NADPH–cytochrome P-450 reductase passes them on to the catalytic enzyme cytochrome P-450.

Monoamine oxidase is a flavoprotein enzyme that is found on the outer membrane of mitochondria. It oxidatively deaminates short-chain monoamines only and it is not part of the DMMS. Adenosine triphosphate (ATP) is involved in transfer of reducing equivalents through the mitochondrial respiratory chain, not the microsomal system.

Anti-Infectives

Note: In the classification of drugs in this and subsequent chapters, prototype drugs are marked with an asterisk.

General Concepts: β-Lactam Antibiotics
- Cell-wall synthesis
  - Inhibition by β-lactam antibiotics
- Autolytic enzyme activity
  - Autolysin-deficient bacteria
- Penicillin-binding proteins (PBPs)
- Mechanisms of resistance
  - Permeability barrier
  - β-Lactamase production

Penicillins
- Natural penicillins
  - Penicillin G*
  - Penicillin V
- Penicillinase-resistant
  - Methacillin
  - Nafcillin
  - Oxacillin
  - Cloxacillin
  - Dicloxacillin
- Aminopenicillins
  - Ampicillin*
  - Amoxicillin
- Extended-spectrum
  - Carbenicillin
  - Ticarcillin
  - Azlocillin
  - Mezlocillin
  - Piperacillin

β-Lactamase Inhibitors
- Clavulanic acid*
- Sulbactam
- Tazobactam

Cephalosporins
- First generation
  - Parenteral use
    - Cefazolin
    - Cephalothin*
    - Cephapirin
    - Cephradine
  - Oral use
    - Cephalexin*
    - Cefadroxil
    - Cephradine
- Second generation
  - Parenteral use
    - Cefuroxime*
    - Cefonicid
    - Cefmetazole
    - Cefoxitin
    - Cefotetan
  - Oral use
    - Cefaclor*
    - Cefuroxime
    - Cefprozil
    - Loracarbef
- Third generation
  - Parenteral use
    - Cefotaxime*
    - Ceftizoxime
    - Cefoperazone
    - Ceftriaxone
  - Oral use
    - Cefixime
    - Cefpodoxime proxetil

- Carbapenems
  - Imipenem-cilastatin
- Monobactams
  - Aztreonam

Miscellaneous Antibiotics
- Primarily against gram-positives
  - Erythromycin*
  - Clarithromycin*
  - Vancomycin*
- Primarily against anaerobes
  - Clindamycin*
  - Metronidazole*
- Primarily against gram-negatives
  - Streptomycin*
  - Gentamicin
  - Tobramycin
  - Amikacin
  - Netilmicin
  - Ciprofloxacin
  - Norfloxacin
  - Enoxacin
  - Ofloxacin
  - Lomefloxacin
- Primarily for *N. gonorrhoeae*
  - Spectinomycin (not an aminoglycoside)

Broad-Spectrum Antimicrobials
- Chloramphenicol*
- Clindamycin
- Metronidazole
- Tetracyclines*
  - Tetracycline
  - Oxytetracycline
  - Demeclocycline
  - Methacycline
  - Doxycycline
  - Minocycline
- Sulfonamides
  - Sulfisoxazole
  - Sulfadiazine*
  - Sulfamethoxazole
  - Sulfamerazine
  - Sulfamethazine
  - Sulfamethizole
  - Sulfameter
  - Sulfadoxine

Trimethoprim*
- Trimethoprim-sulfamethoxazole*

Antituberculosis drugs
- Isoniazid*
- Rifampin*
- Ethambutol*
- Pyrazinamide
- Streptomycin*
- Ethionamide
- Capreomycin
- Kanamycin
- Para-aminosalicylic acid (PAS)

Drugs for leprosy
- Dapsone*
- Clofazimine

Antimycotic drugs
- Amphotericin B*
- Nystatin*
- Flucytosine*
- Griseofulvin*
- Ketoconazole*
- Miconazole
- Butoconazole
- Oxiconazole

Antiviral drugs
- Amantadine*
- Acyclovir*
- Vidarabine
- Trifluridine
- Idoxuridine*
- Ribavirin
- Zidovudine*

Protozoan infections
- Malaria
  - Quinine, mefloquine*
  - Chloroquine*
  - Primaquine*

Proguanil
Pyrimethamine*
Trimethoprim
Sulfonamides
Qinghaosu, artemisinine

Amebiasis
Diloxanide furoate*
Metronidazole*
Tinidazole
Emetine*
Dehydroemetine
Iodoquinol*
Paromomycin
Carbarsone
Chloroquine

Leishmaniasis
Sodium stibogluconate*
Amphotericin B*
Metronidazole*
Allopurinol
Nifurtimox

Trypanosomiasis
Pentamidine
Melarsoprol
Nifurtimox
Suramin

Giardiasis
Metronidazole
Quinacrine
Furazolidone

Trichomoniasis
Metronidazole

Toxoplasmosis
Pyrimethamine-sulfadiazine

Pneumonia caused by *P. carinii*
Trimethoprim-sulfamethoxazole
Pentamidine

Antihelmintics
Mebendazole
Diethylcarbamazine
Pyrantel
Thiabendazole
Piperazine
Quinacrine
Niclosamide
Oxamniquine
Praziquantel

DIRECTIONS: Each question below contains five suggested responses. Select the **one best** response to each question.

43. Kernicterus in newborn or premature infants treated with sulfonamides is due to

(A) enhanced synthesis of bilirubin
(B) displacement of bound bilirubin from albumin
(C) inhibition of bilirubin degradation
(D) inhibition of urinary excretion of bilirubin
(E) deposition of crystalline aggregates in the kidneys

44. Aluminum and calcium salts inhibit the intestinal absorption of which of the following agents?

(A) Isoniazid
(B) Chloramphenicol
(C) Phenoxymethyl penicillin
(D) Erythromycin
(E) Tetracycline

45. The drug used alone for the radical cure or causal prophylaxis of malaria caused by *Plasmodium vivax* or *P. ovale* is

(A) primaquine
(B) pyrimethamine
(C) quinacrine
(D) chloroquine
(E) chloroguanide

46. The quinolone derivative effective against *P. aeruginosa* is

(A) norfloxacin
(B) ciprofloxacin
(C) ofloxacin
(D) enoxacin
(E) lomefloxacin

47. Sulfonamides specifically inhibit which of the following processes?

(A) Conversion of tetrahydrofolic acid to dihydrofolic acid
(B) Conversion of folic acid to folinic acid
(C) Synthesis of DNA
(D) Synthesis of folic acid
(E) Reduction of ribonucleotides

48. The elimination half-life of which of the following tetracyclines remains unchanged when the drug is administered to an anuric patient?

(A) Methacycline
(B) Oxytetracycline
(C) Doxycycline
(D) Tetracycline
(E) None of the above

49. In the treatment of bacterial meningitis in children, the drug of choice is

(A) penicillin G
(B) penicillin VK
(C) erythromycin
(D) procaine penicillin
(E) ceftriaxone

50. In patients with hepatic coma, decreases in the production and absorption of ammonia from the gastrointestinal tract will be beneficial. The antibiotic of choice in this situation would be

(A) neomycin
(B) tetracycline
(C) penicillin G
(D) chloramphenicol
(E) cephalothin

51. Indicate from the diagram below the site of action of penicillinase.

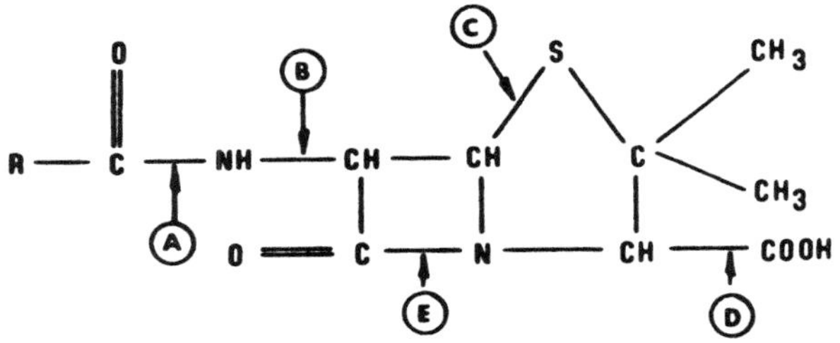

(A) A
(B) B
(C) C
(D) D
(E) E

---

52. Clavulanic acid is important because it

(A) easily penetrates gram-negative microorganisms
(B) is specific for gram-positive microorganisms
(C) is a potent inhibitor of cell wall transpeptidase
(D) inactivates bacterial β-lactamases
(E) has a spectrum of activity similar to that of penicillin G

53. In the treatment of infections caused by *Pseudomonas aeruginosa,* the antimicrobial agent that has proved to be effective is

(A) penicillin G
(B) piperacillin
(C) nafcillin
(D) erythromycin
(E) tetracycline

54. Ethambutol is administered concurrently with other antitubercular drugs in the treatment of tuberculosis in order to

(A) reduce the pain of injection
(B) facilitate penetration of the blood-brain barrier
(C) retard the development of organism resistance
(D) delay excretion of other antitubercular drugs by the kidney
(E) retard absorption after intramuscular injection

55. The most active aminoglycoside against *Mycobacterium tuberculosis* is

(A) streptomycin
(B) amikacin
(C) neomycin
(D) tobramycin
(E) kanamycin

56. The drug used in all types of tuberculosis is

(A) ethambutol
(B) cycloserine
(C) streptomycin
(D) isoniazid
(E) *p*-aminosalicylic acid

57. Chronic candidiasis infections of the gastrointestinal tract and oral cavity are treated *orally* with

(A) amphotericin B
(B) nystatin
(C) miconazole
(D) fluconazole
(E) clotrimazole

58. Isoniazid, one of the most active drugs for the treatment of tuberculosis,

(A) cannot be used with rifampin or ethambutol
(B) works primarily by preventing protein synthesis
(C) possesses toxicities that can be prevented by pyridoxine
(D) is removed from the body unchanged
(E) is rarely met with resistance to its action

59. For the treatment of a patient with *Legionella* pneumonia, the drug of choice would be

(A) penicillin G
(B) chloramphenicol
(C) erythromycin
(D) streptomycin
(E) lincomycin

60. The most effective agent in the treatment of *Rickettsia, Mycoplasma,* and *Chlamydia* infections is

(A) penicillin G
(B) tetracycline
(C) vancomycin
(D) gentamicin
(E) bacitracin

61. The mechanism of action by which pyrantel pamoate is effective for the treatment of hookworm disease is

(A) interference with cell-wall synthesis
(B) interference with cell division
(C) inhibition of neuromuscular transmission
(D) interference with protein synthesis
(E) depletion of membrane lipoproteins

62. Vertigo, inability to perceive termination of movement, and difficulty in sitting or standing without visual clues are some of the toxic reactions that are likely to occur in about 75 percent of patients who

(A) are allergic to penicillin
(B) receive tetracycline therapy
(C) receive amphotericin B therapy
(D) receive streptomycin therapy
(E) receive isoniazid therapy for tuberculosis

63. Amantadine (Symmetrel), a synthetic antiviral agent used prophylactically against influenza A_2, is thought to act by

(A) preventing production of viral capsid protein
(B) preventing virion release
(C) preventing penetration of the virus into the host cell
(D) preventing synthesis of nucleic acid
(E) causing lysis of infected host cells by release of intracellular lysosomal enzymes

64. Streptomycin and other aminoglycosides inhibit bacterial protein synthesis by binding

(A) peptidoglycan units in the cell wall
(B) messenger RNA
(C) DNA
(D) 30S ribosomal particles
(E) RNA polymerase

65. Which of the following statements concerning griseofulvin is true?

(A) It inhibits the growth of dermatophytes
(B) It inhibits synthesis of the cell wall
(C) It inhibits synthesis of the cell membrane
(D) It is used primarily as a short-term drug
(E) It is administered primarily by the parenteral route

66. Which of the following is the most accurate statement concerning the pharmacology of erythromycin?

(A) It binds to the 50S ribosomal subunit at the P binding site
(B) It is classified as an aminoglycoside
(C) It has cross-sensitization to penicillins
(D) It possesses ototoxicity
(E) Transport across the cytoplasmic bacterial membrane is energy-dependent

67. Which of the following cephalosporins would have increased activity against anaerobic bacteria such as *Bacteroides fragilis?*

(A) Cefaclor
(B) Cephalothin
(C) Cephalexin
(D) Cefamandole
(E) Cefoxitin

68. Which one of the following antimicrobial agents is primarily administered topically?

(A) Polymyxin B
(B) Penicillin G
(C) Dicloxacillin
(D) Carbenicillin
(E) Streptomycin

69. Streptomycin is an effective aminoglycoside that

(A) is administered orally
(B) is not significantly metabolized
(C) does not accumulate in patients with renal impairment
(D) is used widely against gram-positive enteric bacteria
(E) is ineffective against tuberculosis

70. Which one of the following statements is correct about vancomycin?

(A) It inhibits cell-wall synthesis
(B) It is primarily effective against gram-negative organisms
(C) It is administered primarily by the oral route
(D) It is the cause of Franconi syndrome
(E) It is the cause of "gray baby syndrome"

71. Which one of the following penicillins is resistant to penicillinase?

(A) Ampicillin
(B) Oxacillin
(C) Carbenicillin
(D) Ticarcillin
(E) Mezlocillin

72. The clinical application of carbenicillin is most accurately reflected by which of the following statements?

(A) It has little activity against gram-negative bacteria
(B) It is ineffective against *Pseudomonas*
(C) It can cause hypokalemic alkalosis
(D) It frequently causes diarrhea
(E) It is resistant to β-lactamase

73. One of the mechanisms associated with bacteria's resistance to penicillin is

(A) ability of bacteria to produce an acid media
(B) bacterial production of lysozymes
(C) alteration of penicillin-binding proteins (PBPs)
(D) increased metabolism of the penicillin
(E) increased renal excretion of penicillins

74. Ketoconazole is a broadly useful antifungal compound that

(A) is usually administered parenterally
(B) possesses androgenic activity
(C) is excellent for infections of the central nervous system
(D) is effective in chronic suppressive therapy for mucocutaneous candidiasis
(E) can cause steroid abnormalities in patients

75. Thiabendazole (Mintezol), a benzimidazole derivative, is an anthelmintic drug used primarily to treat infections caused by

(A) *Ascaris*
(B) *Necator americanus* (hookworm)
(C) *Strongyloides*
(D) *Enterobius vermicularis*
(E) *Taenia saginata* (flatworm)

76. Sulfonamides may cause renal damage that has been shown to be the result of precipitation of crystals in the collecting tubules of the kidney. Predisposing factors to such crystal formation include

(A) low urinary concentration of the drug
(B) high urinary solubility of the drug
(C) a urine pH of 5.0
(D) simultaneous administration of several sulfonamides
(E) administration of the drug parenterally

77. The mechanism of action of chloroquine in *Plasmodium falciparum* malaria is elimination of

(A) secondary tissue schizonts
(B) exoerythrocytic schizonts
(C) the erythrocytic stage
(D) asexual forms
(E) sporozoites

78. The use of chloramphenicol may result in

(A) bone marrow stimulation
(B) phototoxicity
(C) aplastic anemia
(D) staining of teeth
(E) alopecia

79. A drug primarily used in pneumonia caused by *Pneumocystis carinii* is

(A) nifurtimox
(B) penicillin G
(C) metronidazole
(D) pentamidine
(E) carbenicillin

80. A third-generation cephalosporin is

(A) cephalexin
(B) cefoperazone
(C) cefoxitin
(D) cephalothin
(E) cefamandole

81. A fresh case of amebic dysentery is most appropriately treated with metronidazole. An accurate characterization of this drug is that it

(A) is the treatment of choice for asymptomatic carriers of cysts
(B) is poorly absorbed from the intestinal tract
(C) has more severe adverse effects than does emetine
(D) is effective in both the intestinal (luminal) and tissue stages of *Entamoeba histolytica*
(E) is ineffective against trichomoniasis

82. One of the reasons aminoglycosides are frequently combined with other antibiotics to treat certain infections is to

(A) prevent drug interactions
(B) prevent the emergence of resistant bacteria
(C) increase renal excretion
(D) increase oral absorption
(E) decrease systemic toxicities

83. Neuromuscular blockade produced by tubocurarine is potentiated by

(A) neomycin
(B) bacitracin
(C) cephalothin
(D) penicillin
(E) chloramphenicol

84. Chloramphenicol, a completely synthetic antibiotic, is the drug of choice in

(A) symptomatic *Salmonella* infections
(B) brucellosis
(C) urinary tract infection by *Escherichia coli*
(D) cholera
(E) streptococcal pharyngitis

85. In comparing penicillins and cephalosporins, which of the following statements is most valid?

(A) Cephalosporins are only bacteriostatic against multiplying bacteria
(B) Cephalosporins and penicillins have dissimilar mechanisms of activity
(C) Cross-hypersensitivity exists between cephalosporins and penicillins
(D) Cephalosporins are resistant to inactivation by β-lactamase
(E) Cephalosporins are usually administered orally

86. Of the following, the most appropriate statement concerning the reactions caused by aminoglycosides is that these agents

(A) produce ototoxicity
(B) are potent neuromuscular blockers
(C) have little or no effect on kidneys
(D) produce a high incidence of hypersensitivity reactions similar to those of penicillins
(E) produce a high incidence of exfoliated dermatitis

87. A pharmacologic property of amphotericin B is

(A) effective gastrointestinal absorption
(B) usefulness in the treatment of systemic mycoses
(C) binding to DNA
(D) absence of renal toxicity
(E) inhibition of cell-wall synthesis

88. The gray baby syndrome, which is caused by chloramphenicol in the newborn, is

(A) not a serious problem
(B) related to an immature hepatic conjugating mechanism
(C) unrelated to renal function
(D) characterized by life-threatening hyperthermia
(E) associated with hypertension

89. To inhibit the antibacterial activity of sulfonamides, one should administer

(A) acetylsalicylate
(B) folic acid
(C) pantothenic acid
(D) vitamin B_{12}
(E) methotrexate

90. The activity of dihydrofolate reductase is inhibited by

(A) succinylsulfathiazole (Sulfsuxidine)
(B) trimethoprim
(C) sulfamethoxazole (Gantanol)
(D) tetracycline
(E) griseofulvin

91. The mechanism of action of chloramphenicol as an antibiotic is that it

(A) binds to the 30S ribosome subunit
(B) reversibly binds to the 50S ribosome subunit
(C) prevents cell-membrane development
(D) inhibits cell-wall synthesis
(E) inhibits RNAase polymerase

92. The drug of choice for the treatment of *Taenia saginata* (tapeworm) is

(A) praziquantel
(B) ceftriaxone
(C) primaquine
(D) niclosamide
(E) chloroquine

93. The drug of choice for the treatment of *Schistosoma haematobium* is

(A) praziquantel
(B) ceftriaxone
(C) metronidazole
(D) mebendazole
(E) diethylcarbamazine

94. Ampicillin and amoxicillin are in the same group of penicillins. Which of the following statements best characterizes amoxicillin?

(A) It has better oral absorption than does ampicillin
(B) It can be used in penicillinase-producing organisms
(C) It is classified as a broad-spectrum penicillin
(D) It does not cause hypersensitivity reactions
(E) It is effective against *Pseudomonas*

DIRECTIONS: Each numbered question or incomplete statement below is NEGATIVELY phrased. Select the **one best** lettered response.

95. All the following agents are β-lactam antibiotics EXCEPT

(A) penicillins
(B) cephalosporins
(C) monobactams
(D) quinolones
(E) carbapenems

96. All the following are properties of amphotericin B EXCEPT

(A) it can cause renal and liver dysfunctions
(B) it is poorly absorbed via the oral route
(C) it is used for the treatment of systemic fungal infections
(D) it binds to ergosterol to disturb the fungal membrane
(E) it is a potent inhibitor of cell-wall synthesis

97. Extended-spectrum penicillins are correctly described by all the following statements EXCEPT

(A) mezlocillin and piperacillin are drugs in this category
(B) they are effective against gram-negative bacilli
(C) they are susceptible to staphylococcal penicillinase
(D) they are the drugs of choice for "strep" throat
(E) they produce cross-sensitization with the natural penicillins

98. All the following antibiotics inhibit bacterial cell-wall synthesis EXCEPT

(A) bacitracin
(B) cycloserine
(C) cephalothin
(D) vancomycin
(E) polymyxins

99. All the following penicillins are resistant to penicillinase EXCEPT

(A) oxacillin
(B) cloxacillin
(C) ticarcillin
(D) nafcillin
(E) dicloxacillin

100. Quinine, an antimalarial drug, causes all the following EXCEPT

(A) local anesthesia
(B) local destruction of tissue
(C) analgesia
(D) antipyretic effects
(E) hypertension

101. Idoxuridine is a synthetic antiviral agent with all the following properties EXCEPT

(A) a structure containing a halogen atom
(B) activity against DNA viruses
(C) major use in the treatment of herpes simplex keratitis
(D) topical use on the eye
(E) major use in treatment of herpes simplex virus type 2

102. All the following are associated with the use of penicillin EXCEPT

(A) hypersensitization
(B) interstitial nephritis
(C) impaired platelet function
(D) seizures
(E) disulfiram-like reaction

103. All the following statements are true concerning cephalosporins in comparison with penicillins EXCEPT

(A) their structures are closely related
(B) their mechanisms of action are analogous
(C) cephalosporins have an unusually broader antimicrobial spectrum
(D) their hypersensitivity reactions are distinguished by distinct signs and symptoms
(E) cephalosporins can cause bleeding problems related to hypoprothrombinemia

104. All the following statements are associated with the antibiotic methicillin EXCEPT

(A) it causes hypersensitivity
(B) it is administered only orally
(C) it is resistant to penicillinase
(D) it causes interstitial nephritis
(E) it is poorly bound to serum proteins

105. Metronidazole is effective in the treatment of all the following EXCEPT

(A) trichomoniasis in females
(B) asymptomatic trichomoniasis in males
(C) giardiasis
(D) infection with *Bacteroides fragilis*
(E) streptococcal infection

106. Common complications of cephalothin therapy in hospitalized patients include all the following EXCEPT

(A) fever, eosinophilia, and anaphylaxis
(B) superinfection with gram-negative organisms
(C) thrombophlebitis
(D) nephrotoxicity
(E) hemolytic anemia

107. All the following statements are true of acyclovir EXCEPT

(A) it is a nucleoside antiviral drug
(B) it converts to a triphosphate and subsequently inhibits synthesis of viral DNA
(C) it is available topically and orally
(D) it is used against herpes simplex
(E) it is an analogue of purine metabolites

108. By certain changes in the side chain of penicillin structure, the pharmacology is markedly altered. Carbenicillin has all the following properties EXCEPT

(A) it is classified as an aminopenicillin
(B) it is given only parenterally
(C) it is sensitive to penicillinase
(D) it is effective against most gram-negative organisms
(E) in combination with an aminoglycoside, it exhibits increased activity against *Pseudomonas*

DIRECTIONS: Each group of questions below consists of lettered headings followed by a set of numbered items. For each numbered item select the **one** lettered heading with which it is **most** closely associated. Each lettered heading may be used **once, more than once, or not at all**.

Questions 109–111

For each of the antibiotics below, select the appropriate mode of action.

(A) Binds to the 30S ribosome subunit
(B) Inhibits cell-membrane synthesis
(C) Inhibits binding of aminoacyl RNA to the 50S ribosome subunit
(D) Inhibits folic acid reductase
(E) Inhibits production of cell wall
(F) Reversibly binds to the 50S ribosome subunit
(G) Inhibits RNA polymerase
(H) Inhibits synthesis of steroids

109. Streptomycin

110. Erythromycin

111. Penicillin G

Questions 112–114

For each of the parasites below, select the drug that is most effective against it.

(A) Bithionol
(B) Methotrexate
(C) Pyrantel pamoate
(D) Penicillin
(E) Praziquantel
(F) Ceftriaxone
(G) Diethylcarbamazine (Hetrazan)
(H) Primaquine
(I) Niclosamide
(J) Chloroquine

112. *Ascaris lumbricoides* (roundworms)

113. *Wuchereria bancrofti* (filariae)

114. *Fasciola hepatica* (sheep liver flukes)

Questions 115–117

For each of the drugs below, select the most suitable description.

(A) Parenteral penicillin that is resistant to β-lactamase
(B) Oral penicillin that is resistant to β-lactamase
(C) Referred to as an extended-spectrum penicillin
(D) Chemically a cephalosporin
(E) Related to ampicillin but with better oral absorption
(F) Administered intramuscularly and yields prolonged drug levels
(G) Cause of a disulfiram-like reaction
(H) Given parenterally and may cause elevation of serum sodium
(I) Cause of hypothrombinemia

115. Benzathine penicillin G

116. Methicillin

117. Piperacillin

Anti-Infectives

Answers

43. The answer is B. *(DiPalma, 4/e, p 738. Gilman, 8/e, p 1037.)* Sulfonamides should not be used in neonates, especially premature infants, since the drug competes with bilirubin for serum albumin binding. This results in increased levels of free bilirubin, which cause kernicterus. Pregnant women at term also should not receive sulfonamides because of this drug's ability to cross the placenta and enter the fetus in concentrations sufficient to produce toxic effects.

44. The answer is E. *(DiPalma, 4/e, pp 744–745. Gilman, 8/e, p 1119.)* Tetracyclines, as chelating agents, have a high affinity for the divalent cations of calcium and magnesium salts, for iron-containing preparations, for dairy products, and for aluminum hydroxide gels. The chelated complex is insoluble and not absorbed through the mucosa of the gastrointestinal tract. Tetracyclines should be administered before meals to prevent formation of such chelates. Antacids that contain cations of calcium, magnesium, or aluminum should not be administered simultaneously with tetracyclines. These cations do not affect the absorption of the other drugs listed in the question.

45. The answer is A. *(DiPalma, 4/e, pp 778–779. Gilman, 8/e, pp 988–989.)* Primaquine is effective against the extraerythrocytic forms of *P. vivax* and *P. ovale* and is thus of value in a radical cure of malarial infection. It also attacks the sexual forms of the parasite, rendering them incapable of maturation in the mosquito. This makes it valuable in the prevention of the spread of malarial infection.

46. The answer is B. *(DiPalma, 4/e, pp 724–725. Gilman, 8/e, pp 1059–1060.)* Ciprofloxacin is a fluorinated quinolone derivative highly effective against *P. aeruginosa*. Other derivatives in this class have little or no activity toward this organism, although they are effective against other common gram-negative organisms.

47. The answer is D. *(DiPalma, 4/e, p 736. Gilman, 8/e, p 1048.)* Sulfonamides, structural analogues of para-aminobenzoic acid, specifically inhibit the synthesis of folic acid. This in turn leads to inhibition of protein, RNA, and DNA synthesis and to concomitant cessation of growth because folic acid in its cofactor form is required for the synthesis of all these macromolecules. The fact that human cells do not contain folic acid synthetase is the basis for the selective toxicity of the sulfonamides.

48. The answer is C. *(DiPalma, 4/e, p 745. Gilman, 8/e, pp 1121–1122.)* All tetracyclines can produce negative nitrogen balance and increased blood urea nitrogen (BUN) levels. This is of clinical importance in patients with impaired renal function. With the exception of doxycycline, tetracyclines should not be used in patients that are anuric. Doxycycline is excreted by the gastrointestinal tract under these conditions and it will not accumulate in the serum of patients with renal insufficiency.

49. The answer is E. *(DiPalma, 4/e, pp 712–713. Gilman, 8/e, pp 1090–1091.)* Penicillins are rarely used in the treatment of meningitis because of their failure to pass across the blood-brain barrier. Most cephalosporins also have poor penetration into the central nervous system, but the third-generation cephalosporin ceftriaxone is highly effective against *Haemophilus influenzae* meningitis in children.

50. The answer is A. *(Gilman, 8/e, p 1112.)* Neomycin, an aminoglycoside, is not significantly absorbed from the gastrointestinal tract. After oral administration, the intestinal flora is suppressed or modified and the drug is excreted in the feces. This effect of neomycin is used in hepatic coma to decrease the coliform flora, thus decreasing the production of ammonia causing the levels of free nitrogen to decrease in the bloodstream. Other antimicrobial agents—such as tetracycline, penicillin G, chloramphenicol, and cephalothin—do not have the potency of neomycin in causing this effect.

51. The answer is E. *(DiPalma, 4/e, p 696. Gilman, 8/e, pp 1066–1067.)* Penicillinase hydrolyzes the β-lactam ring of penicillin G to form inactive penicillonic acid. Consequently, the antibiotic is ineffective in the therapy of infections caused by penicillinase-producing microorganisms such as staphylococci, bacilli, *Escherichia coli, Pseudomonas aeruginosa,* and *Mycobacterium tuberculosis.*

52. The answer is D. *(DiPalma, 4/e, pp 705–706. Gilman, 8/e, p 1093.)* The antibiotic clavulanic acid is a potent inhibitor of β-lactamases. The mode of inhibition is irreversible. Although clavulanic acid does not effectively inhibit the transpeptidase, it may be used in conjunction with a β-lactamase-sensitive penicillin to potentiate its activity.

53. The answer is B. *(DiPalma, 4/e, pp 704–705. Gilman, 8/e, p 1069.)* Piperacillin is a broad-spectrum, semisynthetic penicillin for parenteral use. Its spectrum of activity includes various gram-positive and gram-negative organisms including *Pseudomonas*. The indications for piperacillin are similar to those for carbenicillin, ticarcillin, and mezlocillin with the primary use being suspected or proven infections caused by *P. aeruginosa*. Penicillin G, nafcillin, erythromycin, and tetracycline are ineffective against *Pseudomonas*.

54. The answer is C. *(DiPalma, 4/e, pp 750–751. Gilman, 8/e, p 1158.)* An important problem in the chemotherapy of tuberculosis is bacterial drug resistance. For this reason, concurrent administration of two or more drugs should be employed to delay the development of drug resistance. Isoniazid (Nydrazid) is often combined with ethambutol (Myambutol) for this purpose. Streptomycin or rifampin (Rifadin) may also be added to the regimen to delay even further the development of drug resistance.

55. The answer is A. *(DiPalma, 4/e, pp 721–722. Gilman, 8/e, p 1153.)* The activity of streptomycin is bactericidal for the tubercle bacillus organism. Other aminoglycosides—such as gentamicin, tobramycin, neomycin, amikacin, and kanamycin—have activity against this organism but are seldom used clinically because of toxicity or development of resistance.

56. The answer is D. *(DiPalma, 4/e, pp 747–748. Gilman, 8/e, pp 1148–1149.)* Isoniazid is an effective tuberculostatic drug. Only actively growing bacilli are susceptible to the bactericidal property of isoniazid. The major action of isoniazid is on the cell wall of the bacillus, where it prevents the synthesis of mycolic acid.

57. The answer is D. *(DiPalma, 4/e, pp 757, 759. Gilman, 8/e, pp 1177–1179.)* Mucocutaneous infections, most commonly *Candida albicans*, involve the moist skin and mucous membranes. Agents used topically include amphotericin B, nystatin, miconazole, and clotrimazole. Ketoconazole and fluconazole are administered orally for treatment of chronic infections.

58. The answer is C. *(DiPalma, 4/e, pp 747–748. Gilman, 8/e, pp 1146–1149.)* Isoniazid is the most widely useful drug in tuberculosis, in combination with rifampin or ethambutol. The mechanism of action of isoniazid involves the inhibition of synthesis of mycolic acids. Isoniazid is metabolized to an acetylated form. Some toxic reactions include peripheral neuritis, insomnia, and restlessness. The peripheral neuritis can be prevented by pretreatment with pyridoxine.

59. The answer is C. *(DiPalma, 4/e, p 730. Gilman, 8/e, pp 1133–1134.)* Erythromycin, a macrolide antibiotic, was initially designed to be used in penicillin-sensitive patients with streptococcal or pneumococcal infections. Erythromycin has become the drug of choice for the treatment of pneumonia caused by *Mycoplasma* and *Legionella.*

60. The answer is B. *(DiPalma, 4/e, pp 743–745. Gilman, 8/e, pp 1123–1124.)* Tetracycline is one of the drugs of choice in the treatment of *Rickettsia, Mycoplasma,* and *Chlamydia* infections. The antibiotics that act by inhibiting cell wall synthesis have no effect on *Mycoplasma* since the organism does not possess a cell wall; penicillin G, vancomycin, and bacitracin will be ineffective. Gentamicin has little or no antimicrobial activity with these organisms.

61. The answer is C. *(DiPalma, 4/e, pp 794–795. Gilman, 8/e, pp 969–970.)* Pyrantel pamoate is an anthelmintic that acts primarily as a depolarizing neuromuscular blocker. In certain worms, a spastic neuromuscular paralysis occurs, resulting in the expulsion of the worms from the intestinal tract of the host. Pyrantel also exerts its effect against parasites via release of acetylcholine and inhibition of cholinesterase.

62. The answer is D. *(DiPalma, 4/e, pp 722–723. Gilman, 8/e, pp 1104–1108.)* Streptomycin and other aminoglycosides can elicit toxic reactions involving both the vestibular and auditory branches of the eighth cranial nerve. Patients receiving an aminoglycoside should be monitored frequently for any hearing impairment owing to the irreversible deafness that may result from its prolonged use. None of the other agents listed in the question adversely affect the function of the eighth cranial nerve.

63. The answer is C. *(DiPalma, 4/e, pp 764, 767. Gilman, 8/e, p 1191.)* Amantadine's mechanism of action is not entirely understood, but it appears to block the attachment of the virus to cells. The drug does not affect penetration and RNA-dependent RNA polymerase activity. Amantadine both reduces the frequency of illness and diminishes the serologic response to influenza infection. The drug has no action, however, on influenza B. As a weak base, amantadine buffers the pH of endosomes, thus blocking the fusion of the viral envelope with the membrane of the endosome.

64. The answer is D. *(DiPalma, 4/e, pp 719–720. Gilman, 8/e, p 1100.)* The bactericidal activity of streptomycin and other aminoglycosides involves a direct action on the 30S ribosomal subunit, the site at which these agents both inhibit protein synthesis and diminish the accuracy of translation of the genetic code. Proteins containing improper sequences of amino acids ("nonsense" proteins) are often nonfunctional.

65. The answer is A. *(DiPalma, 4/e, p 760. Gilman, 8/e, pp 1173–1174.)* Griseofulvin is a potent, orally administered antifungal agent effective against various dermatophytes including *Epidermophyton* and *Trichophyton*. The mechanism of action appears to be related to the interference of nucleic acid synthesis and polymerization. When given for a specific fungal infection, griseofulvin must be continued for 3 to 6 weeks if only hair or skin is involved, but 3 to 6 months if nails are affected.

66. The answer is A. *(DiPalma, 4/e, pp 719, 729–731. Gilman, 8/e, pp 1130–1131.)* Erythromycin is classified as a macrolide that inhibits bacterial protein synthesis by binding to the 50S ribosomal subunit at a site located in the peptidyl-tRNA binding region (P site). This attachment blocks translocation by interfering with the association of peptidyl-tRNA with its binding site after peptide bond formation. Macrolides do not bind to mammalian 80S ribosomes. Unlike the transport of aminoglycosides, the transport of erythromycin across the cytoplasmic bacterial membranes is not energy-dependent.

67. The answer is E. *(DiPalma, 4/e, p 711. Gilman, 8/e, p 1089.)* Cefoxitin and moxalactam are suitable for treating intraabdominal infections. Such infections are caused by mixtures of aerobic and anaerobic gram-negative bacteria like *Bacteroides fragilis*. Cefoxitin alone has been shown to be as effective as the traditional therapy of clindamycin plus gentamicin.

68. The answer is A. *(Gilman, 8/e, pp 1138–1139.)* Polymyxin B is poorly absorbed by the oral route. It is primarily administered by the topical route for the treatment of infections of the skin, mucous membranes, eye, and ear. Penicillin G can be administered both orally and parenterally. Dicloxacillin is only given by the oral route. Carbenicillin and streptomycin are administered only by the parenteral route.

69. The answer is B. *(DiPalma, 4/e, pp 722–723. Gilman, 8/e, pp 1157–1158.)* Streptomycin is poorly absorbed if at all from the gastrointestinal tract. The drug is not broken down in the body and is excreted primarily by the renal route. Therefore, doses must be adjusted in patients with renal disease to prevent accumulation. Streptomycin is very effective against gram-negative enteric bacteria or when there is evidence of sepsis. It is also useful in the treatment of tuberculosis.

70. The answer is A. *(DiPalma, 4/e, pp 716–717. Gilman, 8/e, pp 1138–1140.)* Vancomycin is a bactericidal agent that inhibits cell-wall synthesis. It inhibits the third stage of peptidoglycan synthesis. Virtually all gram-positive bacteria are sensitive to vancomycin; however, the drug has no significant activity against gram-negative organisms. Vancomycin is absorbed poorly from the gastrointestinal tract, so it is administered intravenously. Major toxic reactions include phlebitis, ototoxicity, and nephrotoxicity. Franconi syndrome and "gray baby syndrome" are clinical manifestations of administration of chloramphenicol.

71. The answer is B. *(DiPalma, 4/e, pp 702–703. Gilman, 8/e, pp 1068–1069.)* Oxacillin is resistant to penicillinase; ampicillin, carbenicillin, ticarcillin, and mezlocillin are not. These latter four agents are broad-spectrum penicillins, while oxacillin is generally specific for gram-positive microorganisms. Use of penicillinase-resistant penicillins should be reserved for infections caused by penicillinase-producing staphylococci.

72. The answer is C. *(DiPalma, 4/e, pp 704–706. Gilman, 8/e, pp 1080–1081.)* Carbenicillin resembles ampicillin but has more activity against *Pseudomonas* and *Proteus* organisms than do the standard penicillin G preparations. Carbenicillin is susceptible to penicillinase (β-lactamase), and its activity is lost when hydrolyzed by this enzyme. One of the unusual effects of carbenicillin is its ability to cause a lowering of total body potassium through a renal mechanism, thus leading to hypokalemic alkalosis. Although some gastrointestinal symptoms have been noted with carbenicillin, ampicillin traditionally has been associated with frequent diarrhea.

73. The answer is C. *(DiPalma, 4/e, p 696. Gilman, 8/e, pp 1067–1068.)* Bacterial resistance to β-lactam (penicillin) antibiotics may be due to one or more of the following mechanisms: inability of the drug to penetrate to the target site of its action; alteration of PBPs resulting in reduced affinity for the drug; and inactivation of the drug by bacterial enzymes known as β-lactamases.

74. The answer is D. *(DiPalma, 4/e, pp 760–761. Gilman, 8/e, p 1171.)* Ketoconazole is readily absorbed from the gastrointestinal tract under acidic conditions. It does not penetrate well into the cerebrospinal fluid, which limits its effectiveness in the treatment of infections of the central nervous system. Ketoconazole has antiandrogenic effects by reducing testosterone synthesis. It is very effective in the treatment of chronic mucocutaneous candidiasis. Ketoconazole inhibits steroid biosynthesis by inhibition of cytochrome P-450.

75. The answer is C. *(DiPalma, 4/e, pp 795–796. Gilman, 8/e, pp 972–973.)* Thiabendazole (Mintezol) has been shown to be effective against *Strongyloides,* cutaneous larva migrans, and *Trichuris.* Adverse effects consist of nausea, vertigo, headache, and weakness. Treatment usually involves oral administration for several days. It has been found to be ineffective in *Ascaris, N. americanus, E. vermicularis,* and *T. saginata.*

76. The answer is C. *(DiPalma, 4/e, pp 738–739. Gilman, 8/e, pp 1047–1057.)* Precipitation of sulfonamide crystals may form concentrations that injure the tubular epithelium or the epithelium of the pelvis of the kidney and obstruct the flow of urine. The crystallization is more frequently observed if the solubility of the drug in the urine is low, the pH of the urine is low, or the concentration of the drug in the urine is high. Simultaneous administration of several sulfonamides, each at less than half its normal concentration, permits an adequate bacteriostatic blood concentration to be reached without the risk of renal damage independent of the route of administration.

77. The answer is C. *(DiPalma, 4/e, pp 772–773. Gilman, 8/e, pp 981–982.)* Chloroquine is a 4-aminoquinoline derivative that selectively concentrates in parasitized red blood cells. It is a weak base, and its alkalinizing effect on the acid vesicle of the parasite effectively destroys the viability of the parasite.

78. The answer is C. *(DiPalma, 4/e, p 742. Gilman, 8/e, pp 1127–1129.)* Hematologic toxicity is by far the most important adverse effect of chloramphenicol. The toxicity consists of two types: bone marrow depression (common) and aplastic anemia (rare). Chloramphenicol can produce a potentially fatal toxic reaction, the gray baby syndrome, caused by diminished ability of neonates to conjugate chloramphenicol with resultant high serum concentrations. Tetracyclines produce staining of the teeth and phototoxicity.

79. The answer is D. *(DiPalma, 4/e, p 772. Gilman, 8/e, pp 1011–1013.)* Both trimethoprim-sulfamethoxazole and pentamidine are effective in pneumonia caused by *P. carinii.* This protozoal disease usually occurs in immunodeficient patients such as those with AIDS. Nifurtimox is effective in trypanosomiasis and metronidazole in amebiasis and leishmaniasis, as well as in anaerobic bacterial infections. Penicillins are not considered drugs of choice for this particular disease state.

80. The answer is B. *(DiPalma, 4/e, p 707. Gilman, 8/e, pp 1085–1092.)* The cephalosporins are generally divided into three major categories that have been labeled first, second, and third generations. The cephalosporins are listed in one of these categories according to the spectrum of activity. The first generation includes cephalexin, cephalothin, and cefazolin; the second generation cefaclor and cefoxitin; and the third generation cefoperazone, cefotaxime, and ceftriaxone.

81. The answer is D. *(DiPalma, 4/e, pp 734–736. Gilman, 8/e, pp 1002–1005.)* Metronidazole is not preferred for use against asymptomatic carriers of cysts because it is rapidly absorbed from the intestine; luminal drugs, such as iodoquinol or diloxanide furoate, are preferred, either alone or in combination with metronidazole. Metronidazole is much less toxic than emetine, which had been frequently used in the past. Both the luminal and tissue stages of the ameba are susceptible to metronidazole.

82. The answer is B. *(DiPalma, 4/e, pp 722–723. Gilman, 8/e, pp 1098–1113.)* Aminoglycosides are combined with other antibiotics to increase their antibiotic activity (synergy) and also to decrease the emergence of resistant organisms, especially gram-negative organisms. Generally the combination of two differently acting antibiotics increases the antimicrobial spectrum. The ability of the aminoglycosides to be absorbed orally is not enhanced by combination with other antibiotics nor are there any significant drug interactions or a decrease in potential systemic toxicities.

83. The answer is A. *(DiPalma, 4/e, p 176. Gilman, 8/e, pp 1112–1113.)* Streptomycin, colistin, lincomycin, and clindamycin—in addition to neomycin listed in the question—have also been demonstrated to exert neuromuscular blocking effects that are synergistic with competitive blocking agents such as ether or tubocurarine. This effect is of clinical importance when these antibiotics are administered in large doses intravenously or intraperitoneally.

84. The answer is A. *(DiPalma, 4/e, p 742. Gilman, 8/e, pp 1125–1130.)* Chloramphenicol is the drug of choice in symptomatic *Salmonella* infection (typhoid fever) and also in *Haemophilus influenzae* meningitis in small children, especially when the strain is resistant to ampicillin. Tetracyclines are the drugs of choice for the treatment of brucellosis and cholera. Chloramphenicol may be used in the treatment of brucellosis, however, if tetracycline is contraindicated. Ordinary urinary tract infection and pharyngitis should be treated initially with penicillin.

85. The answer is C. *(DiPalma, 4/e, p 708. Gilman, 8/e, pp 1085–1092.)* Both cephalosporins and penicillins contain a β-lactam ring, and both drugs are sensitive to inactivation by β-lactamase to varying degrees. The mechanisms of action of the two antibiotics are similar: cross-linking of D-alanyl-D-alanine of the peptidoglycan in the formation of bacterial cell walls is inhibited. Cross-allergenicity presumably occurs on the basis of hypersensitivity to similar breakdown products. The majority of the cephalosporins are administered parenterally.

86. The answer is A. *(DiPalma, 4/e, pp 722–723. Gilman, 8/e, pp 1098–1113.)* All the aminoglycosides are potentially toxic to both branches of the eighth cranial nerve. The evidence indicates that the sensory receptor portions of the inner ear are affected rather than the nerve itself. Nephrotoxicity may develop during or after the use of an aminoglycoside. It is generally more common in the elderly when there is preexisting renal dysfunction. In most patients renal function gradually improves after discontinuation of therapy. Aminoglycosides rarely cause neuromuscular blockade that can lead to progressive flaccid paralysis and potential fatal respiratory arrest. Hypersensitivity and dermatologic reactions occasionally occur following use of aminoglycosides.

87. The answer is B. *(DiPalma, 4/e, pp 757–759. Gilman, 8/e, pp 1165–1168.)* Amphotericin B is poorly absorbed from the gastrointestinal tract. The agent's antifungal activity is contingent upon binding of the drug to a sterol moiety present in the membranes of sensitive fungi, which changes the membranes' permeability. Over 80 percent of patients given amphotericin B develop decreased renal function and abnormal urinary sediments. The side effects can be so serious that amphotericin B is restricted to the treatment of severe systemic fungal infections.

88. The answer is B. *(DiPalma, 4/e, p 742. Gilman, 8/e, pp 1125–1130.)* The often fatal gray baby syndrome of chloramphenicol toxicity consists of abdominal distention; vasomotor collapse; diarrhea; rapid, irregular respirations progressing to flaccidity; ashen-gray color (owing to pallid cyanosis); and hypothermia. It is related to the failure of chloramphenicol to be conjugated with glucuronic acid. Neonates have insufficient glucuronyltransferase for conjugation and inadequately developed renal mechanisms for effective excretion of the unconjugated drug.

89. The answer is B. *(DiPalma, 4/e, pp 737–738. Gilman, 8/e, pp 1047–1057.)* The mechanism of action of sulfonamides is thought to be through competitive antagonism of *p*-aminobenzoic acid, the utilization of which by bacteria is essential to synthesis of folic acid. An excess of folic or *p*-aminobenzoic acid will overcome the bacteriostatic effect of sulfonamides. Bacteria that do not need folic acid or can use preformed folic acid are not affected by sulfonamides. Methotrexate inhibits folic acid production and would not interfere with the sulfonamide antimicrobial activity.

90. The answer is B. *(DiPalma, 4/e, p 738. Gilman, 8/e, pp 1054–1057, 1118, 1173.)* The diaminopyrimidines trimethoprim and pyrimethamine are selective inhibitors of dihydrofolate reductase; they have less of an effect on dihydrofolate reductase obtained from mammalian sources. The combination of a diaminopyrimidine and a sulfonamide is synergistic. The combination of trimethoprim and sulfamethoxazole results in inhibition of the activity of dihydrofolate reductase by trimethoprim and inhibition of bacterial synthesis of dihydrofolic acid by the competition between *p*-aminobenzoic acid and sulfamethoxazole. Tetracycline inhibits production of bacterial proteins; griseofulvin interferes with synthesis of nucleic acid.

91. The answer is B. *(DiPalma, 4/e, pp 740–741. Gilman, 8/e, pp 1125–1126.)* Chloramphenicol inhibits protein synthesis in bacteria and, to a lesser extent, in eukaryotic cells. The drug binds reversibly to the 50S ribosomal subunit and prevents attachment of aminoacyl-tRNA to its binding site. The amino acid substrate is unavailable for peptidyl transferase and peptide bond formation.

92. The answer is D. *(DiPalma, 4/e, pp 788, 792–793. Gilman, 8/e, pp 965–966.)* Niclosamide is a halogenated salicylanilide derivative. It exerts its effect against cestodes by inhibition of mitochondrial oxidative phosphorylation in the parasites. The mechanism of action is also related to its inhibition of glucose and oxygen uptake in the parasite.

93. The answer is A. *(DiPalma, 4/e, pp 793–794. Gilman, 8/e, pp 967–969.)* Praziquantel is a broad-spectrum anthelmintic agent. It appears to kill the adult schistosome by increasing the permeability of the cell membranes of the parasite to calcium and consequent influx of calcium ions. This causes increased muscle contraction followed by paralysis.

94. The answer is A. *(DiPalma, 4/e, pp 703–704. Gilman, 8/e, pp 1078–1079.)* Amoxicillin is classified as an aminopenicillin along with ampicillin. Because it is less affected than ampicillin by the presence of food, it has a superior absorption in the gastrointestinal tract. It is sensitive to penicillinase and has a narrow spectrum of activity toward certain gram-positive and gram-negative organisms, but not *Pseudomonas*. Since it is in the penicillin family, hypersensitivity reactions are a possibility.

95. The answer is D. *(DiPalma, 4/e, pp 693–695. Gilman, 8/e, pp 1065–1097.)* β-Lactam antibiotics include penicillins, cephalosporins, monobactams, and carbapenems. All have a four-membered β-lactam ring that is essential for their antibacterial activity. Quinolones are fluorinated derivatives with no relationship chemically to the β-lactam antibiotics.

96. The answer is E. *(DiPalma, 4/e, pp 757–759. Gilman, 8/e, pp 1165–1168.)* Amphotericin B disturbs the permeability and transport mechanisms of membranes by binding to ergosterol in the membrane. It is poorly absorbed via the oral route and must be given parenterally for the treatment of systemic fungal infections. In therapeutic concentrations, amphotericin B has the potential of causing both renal and liver damage, and the dose must be reduced when these toxicities develop. It has little or no activity in cell-wall synthesis.

97. The answer is D. *(DiPalma, 4/e, pp 704–705. Gilman, 8/e, p 1069.)* The extended-spectrum penicillins, which include mezlocillin, azlocillin, and piperacillin, have a broad spectrum of activity against gram-negative bacilli. All are susceptible to staphylococcal penicillinase and must be administered parenterally since they are not absorbed from the gastrointestinal tract. Major toxicity includes the penicillin hypersensitization reaction. They are used only in severe infections that do not respond to natural penicillins.

98. The answer is E. *(DiPalma, 4/e, pp 693–694. Gilman, 8/e, pp 1066, 1139–1140.)* Bacitracin, cycloserine, cephalothin, and vancomycin inhibit cell-wall synthesis and produce bacteria susceptible to environmental conditions. Polymyxins disrupt the structural integrity of the cytoplasmic membranes by acting as cationic detergents. On contact with the drug, the permeability of the membrane changes.

99. The answer is C. *(DiPalma, 4/e, pp 702–704. Gilman, 8/e, pp 1075–1077.)* Ticarcillin resembles carbenicillin and has a high degree of potency against *Pseudomonas* and *Proteus* organisms but is broken down by penicillinase produced by various bacteria, including most staphylococci. Oxacillin, cloxacillin, nafcillin, and dicloxacillin are all resistant to penicillinase and are effective against staphylococci.

100. The answer is E. *(DiPalma, 4/e, pp 776–777. Gilman, 8/e, pp 991–993.)* Quinine has analgesic and antipyretic properties similar to those of the salicylates. When applied locally, quinine has a local anesthetic action in which it briefly stimulates and then paralyzes sensory neurons. Because of its nature as protoplasmic poison, local destruction of tissue often results, which prolongs its action for weeks or months. When administered intravenously, quinine causes hypotension similar to that of its isomer quinidine.

101. The answer is E. *(DiPalma, 4/e, pp 764–765. Gilman, 8/e, p 1188.)* Idoxuridine is a halogenated derivative of deoxyuridine. Its major action is on the DNA viruses, with little or no effect on RNA viruses. Its major use is in the treatment of herpes simplex keratitis, where it is usually used topically on the eye. When used topically, it may cause local irritation, photophobia, and occlusion of the lacrimal duct. Although effective against herpes simplex keratitis, idoxuridine is unresponsive to other herpes infections, including herpes simplex virus type 2 and varicella-zoster virus.

102. The answer is E. *(DiPalma, 4/e, pp 699–670. Gilman, 8/e, p 1091.)* Allergic reactions are the main adverse effects encountered with the use of the penicillins. Sensitization is usually the result of previous treatment with a penicillin. Penicillins are not nephrotoxic; however, allergic interstitial nephritis may occur, particularly with methicillin. Hematologic reactions caused by penicillins are rare, but high concentrations may impair platelet function, resulting in prolongation of bleeding time. Seizures may develop when high doses of penicillins are given in the presence of renal insufficiency. Intolerance of alcohol (disulfiram-like reaction) has been noted only with certain cephalosporins.

103. The answer is D. *(DiPalma, 4/e, pp 706–714. Gilman, 8/e, pp 1085–1092.)* Cephalosporins and penicillins have similar structures, penicillins having a penicillanic acid and the cephalosporins a cephalosporinic acid moiety. Both groups of antimicrobials inhibit the transpeptidase enzyme necessary for cross-linking. It appears that the mechanism is not totally identical for every drug for every bacterial species. Cephalosporins have a greater overall activity against gram-negative organisms than do the penicillin G–type compounds. The hypersensitivity reactions associated with the penicillins and the cephalosporins appear to be identical in signs and symptoms. There is a cross-over sensitivity between the penicillins and cephalosporins that must be considered when a patient is sensitive to either of these antibiotics.

104. The answer is B. *(DiPalma, 4/e, pp 702–703. Gilman, 8/e, p 1075.)* Methicillin is classified as a penicillinase-resistant penicillin that is acid-labile and therefore not useful for oral administration. Major adverse reactions include penicillin hypersensitivity and interstitial nephritis. With the exception of methicillin, which is 35 percent bound to serum proteins, all penicillinase-resistant penicillins are highly bound to plasma proteins.

105. The answer is E. *(DiPalma, 4/e, pp 735–736. Gilman, 8/e, pp 1002–1003.)* Metronidazole is a low-molecular-weight compound that penetrates all tissues and fluids of the body. Metronidazole's spectrum of activity is limited largely to anaerobic bacteria—including *B. fragilis*—and certain protozoa. It is considered to be the drug of choice for trichomoniasis in females and carrier states in males as well as intestinal infections with *Giardia lamblia*.

106. The answer is E. *(DiPalma, 4/e, pp 707–708. Gilman, 8/e, p 1091.)* In about 5 percent of the patients receiving cephalothin, a hypersensitivity reaction develops that is characterized by fever, eosinophilia, serum sickness, rash, and anaphylaxis. A positive Coombs' test result is also frequent but is seldom associated with hemolytic anemia. Thrombophlebitis with intravenous administration of cephalothin is almost universal. Superinfection by cephalothin-resistant gram-negative bacilli has been noted by several observers. The cephalosporins have also been implicated as potentially nephrotoxic agents.

107. The answer is E. *(DiPalma, 4/e, pp 763–764. Gilman, 8/e, pp 1184–1186.)* Acyclovir is a nucleoside analogue of the pyrimidine guanosine. The mechanism of activity involves its conversion to a triphosphate and subsequent inhibition of synthesis of viral DNA. Its activity is highly selective. Acyclovir is available for topical, oral, and intravenous administration and is highly effective against herpes simplex, varicella-zoster, and Epstein-Barr viruses.

108. The answer is A. *(DiPalma, 4/e, pp 704–705. Gilman, 8/e, pp 1080–1081.)* Carbenicillin has a carboxyl group on the side chain and thus is not an aminopenicillin. It is classified as an extended-spectrum penicillin with a wide range of activity against anaerobic gram-negative organisms. It is susceptible to staphylococcal penicillinase organisms. When given with aminoglycosides, a synergistic activity will occur against many isolates of *P. aeruginosa.*

109–111. The answers are 109-A, 110-C, 111-E. *(DiPalma, 4/e, pp 694–695, 721, 729, 743. Katzung, 6/e, pp 671–679.)* Bacterial cells differ from mammalian cells in having a rigid cell wall, which actually forms a compression jacket. The internal osmotic pressure is very high and damage to the cell wall results in bursting of the bacterium. Cephalosporins, penicillins, vancomycin, and ristocetin all inhibit cell-wall synthesis. In particular, penicillins and cephalosporins block the final step in cell-wall synthesis by inhibiting transpeptidase enzymes.

Erythromycin, lincomycin, tetracyclines, and aminoglycoside antibiotics such as amikacin, gentamicin, kanamycin, neomycin, and streptomycin exert their antibacterial action through inhibition of protein synthesis. Erythromycin inhibits binding of aminoacyl tRNAs to the 50S ribosome subunit. Aminoglycosides bind to the 30S subunit as does tetracycline.

Other antibiotics—such as amphotericin B, colistin, nystatin, and polymyxins—inhibit bacteria by disrupting the cellular membrane.

112–114. The answers are 112-C, 113-G, 114-A. *(DiPalma, 4/e, pp 788–790. Katzung, 6/e, pp 804–819.)* Pinworm infestation should be treated with pyrantel in conjunction with rigid standards of personal hygiene. Pyrantel is also the drug of choice against *Ascaris lumbricoides*. A single dose of 11 mg/kg, to a maximum of 1 g, is sufficient.

Filariasis is effectively treated with diethylcarbamazine, a piperazine derivative, which both suppresses and, in most cases, cures the infection. The drug is inactive against *Wuchereria bancrofti* in vitro. However, in vivo activity appears to be due to a sensitization of the microfilaria to phagocytosis by the fixed macrophages of the reticuloendothelial system.

Bithionol has been found useful in the treatment of infection by the sheep liver fluke *Fasciola hepatica* and the lung fluke *Paragonimus kellicotti*. Treatment usually involves the oral administration of 40 to 50 mg/kg, in divided doses on alternate days, for a total of 10 to 15 doses. Chloroquine in large doses has also been successful in the therapy of infection by lung flukes.

115–117. The answers are 115-F, 116-A, 117-C. *(DiPalma, 4/e, pp 700–705. Katzung, 6/e, pp 680–690.)* Because of its long duration of action, benzathine penicillin G is given as a single injection of 1.2 million units intramuscularly every 3 or 4 weeks for the treatment of syphilis. This persistence of action reduces the need for repeated injections, costs, and local trauma. Benzathine penicillin G is also administered for group A, beta-hemolytic streptococcal pharyngitis and pyoderma.

Methicillin is a β-lactamase-resistant (penicillinase-resistant) penicillin that is acid-labile but must be administered by the parenteral route. It is effective against nearly all strains of *Staphylococcus aureus*. Methicillin is much more effective against penicillinase-producing strains than is penicillin G.

Piperacillin along with mezlocillin and azlocillin is commonly referred to as an extended-spectrum penicillin because of its broad spectrum of activity. It is particularly effective against *Klebsiella* and *Pseudomonas*. Piperacillin is available as a powder for solubilization and injection.

Cancer Chemotherapy and Immunology

Plant derivatives
- Etoposide
- Teniposide
- Vincristine sulfate*
- Vinblastine sulfate
- Paclitaxel

Miscellaneous
- Interferon alpha-2a, alpha-2b, alpha-n3*
- Levamisole HCl*
- Altretamine
- Hydroxyurea
- BCG intravesical
- Mitotane
- Asparaginase*

Radiopharmaceuticals
- Sodium iodide ^{131}I*
- Sodium phosphate ^{32}P

Immunopharmacologic Drugs
- Cytotoxic
  - Azathioprine*
  - Cyclophosphamide
  - Vincristine
  - Methotrexate
  - Cytarabine
- Specific T-cell inhibitor
  - Cyclosporine*
- Hormonal
  - Prednisone*
  - Other corticosteroids
- Antibodies
  - Antilymphocyte globulin (ALG)
  - Muromonab-CD_3
  - Rh_o(D) immune globulin

DIRECTIONS: Each question below contains five suggested responses. Select the **one best** response to each question.

118. The most effective drug for immunosuppression of rejection of the allografted kidney is

(A) azathioprine (Imuran)
(B) cyclosporine (Sandimmune)
(C) 5-fluorouracil (5-FU, Adrucil)
(D) cyclophosphamide (Cytoxan)
(E) vincristine (Oncovin)

119. The phase of the cell cycle that is resistant to most chemotherapeutic agents and requires increased dosage to obtain a response is

(A) M phase
(B) G_2 phase
(C) S phase
(D) G_0 phase
(E) G_1 phase

120. A nucleophilic attack on DNA that causes the disruption of base pairing occurs as a result of administration of

(A) cyclophosphamide (Cytoxan)
(B) fluorouracil (5-FU, Adrucil)
(C) methotrexate
(D) prednisone
(E) thioguanine

121. The antineoplastic chemotherapeutic agent that is classified as an alkylating agent is

(A) thioguanine
(B) busulfan (Myleran)
(C) bleomycin (Blenoxane)
(D) vincristine (Oncovin)
(E) tamoxifen (Nolvadex)

122. Which of the following is a chemotherapeutic drug that possesses a mechanism of action involving alkylation?

(A) Cyclophosphamide (Cytoxan)
(B) Methotrexate
(C) Tamoxifen (Nolvadex)
(D) Fluorouracil (5-FU, Adrucil)
(E) Bleomycin (Blenoxane)

123. Which one of the following statements is correct about antimetabolites?

(A) They are structural analogues of naturally occurring substances
(B) They are nontoxic
(C) They do not interfere with metabolic processes
(D) Procarbazine is an example
(E) They have little or no effect on cell proliferation

124. Cardiotoxicity limits the clinical usefulness of which one of the following antitumor antibiotics?

(A) Dactinomycin (Cosmegen)
(B) Doxorubicin (Adriamycin)
(C) Bleomycin (Blenoxane)
(D) Cisplatin (Platinol)
(E) Vincristine (Oncovin)

125. Binding to the enzyme dihydrofolate reductase is the mechanism of action for

(A) procarbazine (Matulane)
(B) paclitaxel (Taxol)
(C) methotrexate
(D) ifosfamide
(E) cladribine (Leustatin)

126. Which of the following is considered to be the effective mechanism of action of the vinca alkaloids?

(A) Inhibition of the function of microtubules
(B) Damage and prevention of repair of DNA
(C) Inhibition of DNA synthesis
(D) Inhibition of protein synthesis
(E) Inhibition of purine synthesis

DIRECTIONS: Each numbered question or incomplete statement below is NEGATIVELY phrased. Select the **one best** lettered response.

127. The tumor LEAST susceptible to "cell cycle–specific" anticancer agents is

(A) acute lymphoblastic leukemia
(B) acute granulocytic leukemia
(C) Burkitt's lymphoma
(D) adenocarcinoma of the colon
(E) choriocarcinoma

128. A 32-year-old cancer patient, who has smoked two packs of cigarettes a day for 10 years, presents a decreased pulmonary function test. Physical examination and chest x-rays suggest preexisting pulmonary disease. All the following drugs may be prescribed EXCEPT

(A) vinblastine (Velban)
(B) doxorubicin (Adriamycin)
(C) mithramycin (Mitracin)
(D) bleomycin (Blenoxane)
(E) cisplatin (Platinol)

129. All the following are cell cycle–specific (CCS) agents EXCEPT

(A) mercaptopurine (6-MP, Purinethol)
(B) fluorouracil (5-FU, Adrucil)
(C) bleomycin (Blenoxane)
(D) busulfan (Myleran)
(E) vincristine (Oncovin)

130. All the following statements regarding the chemotherapy of cancer are valid EXCEPT

(A) 50 percent of all newly diagnosed cancer patients will be cured of their disease
(B) chemotherapy is the only treatment that can effectively treat systemic disease
(C) chemotherapy only kills cancer cells and not normal dividing cells
(D) chemotherapy possesses numerous side effects, such as nausea, vomiting, and suppression of bone marrow
(E) new agents are cell cycle–specific

131. Paclitaxel (Taxol), an agent extracted from the yew tree, has all the following actions and uses EXCEPT

(A) it promotes premature cell division
(B) it can cause neutropenia
(C) it causes disorganized microtubule bundles
(D) it is used to treat metastatic breast cancer
(E) it is a competitive inhibitor at the estrogen receptor

132. Alkylating agents, perhaps the most useful agents in cancer chemotherapy, have all the following actions EXCEPT

(A) they are able to form covalent bonds with nucleophilic sites on nucleic acids
(B) they possess little or no toxicity in the host
(C) they are cytotoxic owing to their activity against DNA
(D) they are able to form a positive carbonium ion
(E) they can affect any part of the cell cycle

133. Allopurinol, an agent useful in gout, also has all the following useful actions in cancer chemotherapy EXCEPT

(A) it inhibits the metabolism of 6-mercaptopurine
(B) it increases the antineoplastic action of 6-mercaptopurine
(C) it inhibits xanthine oxidase
(D) it decreases serum uric acid levels
(E) it possesses uricosuric activity

134. Cyclosporines as effective anti-immune agents have all the following mechanisms of action EXCEPT

(A) they cross cell membranes easily
(B) they bind to a family of intracellular proteins called *cyclophilins*
(C) they inhibit the production of interleukin 2 (IL-2) by helper T cells
(D) they are cytotoxic and depress bone marrow
(E) active biotransformation of cyclosporine is by cytochrome P-450

135. Azathioprine is correctly characterized by all the following statements EXCEPT

(A) it is a prodrug
(B) it has little action on an established graft rejection
(C) it is poorly absorbed in the GI tract
(D) it has a nonselective action in the suppression of lymphoid cells
(E) it greatly increases the susceptibility of the patient to intercurrent infections

136. All the following statements correctly characterize fludarabine (Fludara) EXCEPT

(A) it is a purine derivative
(B) the triphosphate of fludarabine inhibits DNA polymerase
(C) it is effective in nondividing cells
(D) its primary toxicity is myelosuppression
(E) it is biotransformed by xanthine oxidase

137. Glucocorticoids perform all the following immunosuppressive actions EXCEPT

(A) decrease the concentration of antibodies in the circulation
(B) inhibit the synthesis of prostaglandins and leukotrienes
(C) lyse T cells
(D) increase catabolism of gamma G globulin (IgG) on continuous administration
(E) diminish the ability to withstand infections and heal wounds

138. Cyclosporine (Sandimmune) has all the following pharmacologic and toxicologic actions EXCEPT

(A) it is a specific T-cell inhibitor
(B) it has 11 amino acids arranged in a cyclic structure
(C) it crosses cellular membranes easily
(D) it lacks nephrotoxicity
(E) it can cause hyperplasia of gums

139. Drugs classified as immunostimulants include all the following EXCEPT

(A) interferon alpha
(B) aldesleukin
(C) muromonab-CD3
(D) sargramostim
(E) filgrastim

140. Levamisole is an unusual cancer chemotherapeutic agent. It has all the following attributes EXCEPT

(A) anthelmintic properties
(B) immunostimulation
(C) effectiveness in colon cancer with 5-fluorouracil
(D) metallic taste
(E) inhibition of monocyte chemotaxis

DIRECTIONS: Each group of questions below consists of lettered headings followed by a set of numbered items. For each numbered item select the **one** lettered heading with which it is **most** closely associated. Each lettered heading may be used **once, more than once, or not at all.**

Questions 141–143

For each of the drugs below, select the characteristic with which it is most likely to be associated.

(A) Used in treatment of Hodgkin's lymphoma
(B) Classified as an alkylating agent and orally administered
(C) Retained specifically in beta cells of the islets of Langerhans
(D) Used as a single agent against malignant melanoma
(E) Classified as an antitumor antibiotic and results in a high incidence of bone marrow suppression
(F) Used in treatment of breast cancer
(G) Classified as a vinca alkaloid
(H) Used in malignant hypercalcemia
(I) Used in hairy cell leukemia
(J) Derived from hydrazine

141. Streptozocin

142. Dacarbazine

143. Mitomycin (Mutamycin)

Questions 144–146

For each of the indications below, select the correct drug.

(A) Allopurinol (Zyloprim)
(B) Asparaginase (Elspar)
(C) Methotrexate
(D) Streptozocin (Zanosar)
(E) Mercaptopurine (6-MP, Purinethol)
(F) Azathioprine (Imuran)
(G) Pentostatin (Nipent)
(H) Leucovorin
(I) BCG vaccine

144. Severe active rheumatoid arthritis

145. Renal allografts

146. Bladder cancer

Questions 147–149

For each of the drugs below, select the adverse reaction with which it is most closely associated.

(A) Aseptic hemorrhagic cystitis
(B) Cardiotoxicity
(C) Nephrotoxicity
(D) Oral and GI ulceration
(E) Exfoliative dermatitis
(F) Peripheral neuropathy
(G) Convulsions
(H) Pancreatitis
(I) Coma

147. Fluorouracil (5-FU, Adrucil)

148. Asparaginase (Elspar)

149. Procarbazine (Matulane)

Questions 150–152

For each of the chemotherapeutic agents below, choose the phase of the cell cycle at which it is most likely to act.

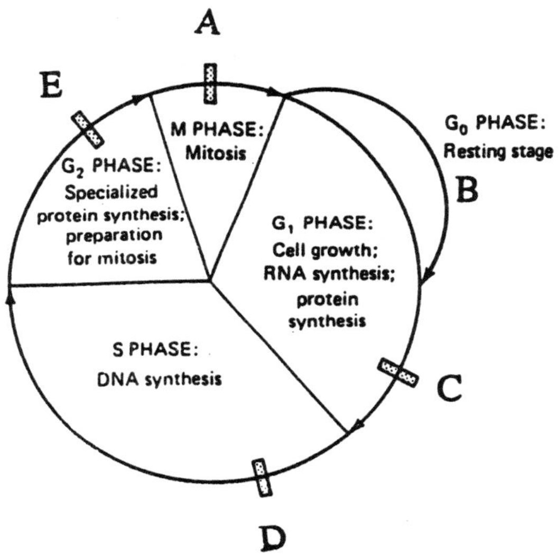

150. Busulfan (Myleran)

151. Dactinomycin (Cosmegen)

152. Dacarbazine

Cancer Chemotherapy and Immunology

Answers

118. The answer is B. *(DiPalma, 4/e, pp 681–683. Gilman, 8/e, pp 1270, 1586.)* Cyclosporine is the preferred agent because it is a specific T-cell inhibitor and its success rate in protecting against rejection is considerably better than that of any other agent. All the other agents in the question are cytotoxic. Because of the severe adverse reactions with cyclosporine, it is used in conjunction with azathioprine, which reduces the required dose. Prednisone is also used in conjunction with cyclosporine.

119. The answer is D. *(AMA Drug Evaluations Annual, 1993, p 1938. DiPalma, 4/e, pp 653–655.)* There are various phases described for the cell cycle. The M phase is the period of cell division (mitosis). Following the M phase a cell may enter either the G_1 phase or G_0 phase. The G_1 phase of the cell cycle is associated with cell growth, RNA synthesis, and protein synthesis. The G_0 phase is the resting or dormant stage. No cell division takes place, although the cells are still capable of undergoing mitosis. This phase of the cell cycle is the most resistant to chemotherapeutic agents and may require a high dosage of the chemotherapeutic agent because most cancer drugs produce their lethal effect on cells that are actively involved in division. The S phase of the cell cycle involves DNA synthesis, and cells that are in the G_2 phase show the synthesis of specialized proteins in preparation for cell replication.

120. The answer is A. *(DiPalma, 4/e, pp 665–666. Gilman, 8/3, p 1210.)* Cyclophosphamide (Cytoxan), an alkylating agent, reacts with purine and pyrimidine bases of DNA to form bridges and dimers. These products interfere with DNA replication. 5-Fluorouracil, methotrexate, and 6-thioguanine are antimetabolites, and the steroid prednisone has some tumor-suppressive effects.

121. The answer is B. *(DiPalma, 4/e, p 657. Gilman, 8/e, pp 1205–1207, 1220.)* Busulfan is an alkylating agent that, in contrast to other alkylators, is an alkylsulfonate. Thioguanine is a purine antimetabolite. Bleomycin is classified as a chemotherapeutic antibiotic and vincristine is a vinca alkaloid. Tamoxifen is an antiestrogen hormone.

122. The answer is A. *(DiPalma, 4/e, p 657. Gilman, 8/e, pp 1205–1207.)* Cyclophosphamide is classified as a polyfunctional alkylating drug that transfers its alkyl groups to cellular components. The cytotoxic effect of this agent is directly associated with the alkylation of components of DNA. Methotrexate and fluorouracil are classified as antimetabolites that block intermediary metabolism to inhibit cell proliferation. Tamoxifen is an antiestrogen compound. Bleomycin is classified as an antibiotic chemotherapeutic agent.

123. The answer is A. *(DiPalma, 4/e, pp 656–663. Katzung, 6/e, pp 832–835.)* Antimetabolites are structural analogues of naturally occurring substances. They interfere with various metabolic processes and disrupt cell function and proliferation. These drugs may act in two ways: (1) by incorporation into the metabolic pathway and formation of a false metabolite that is nonfunctional, or (2) by inhibition of the catalytic function of an enzyme or enzyme system. Procarbazine is classified not as an antimetabolite but as an alkylating agent.

124. The answer is B. *(DiPalma, 4/e, pp 667–669. Gilman, 8/e, pp 1238–1239, 1250.)* Dactinomycin's major toxicities include stomatitis, alopecia, and bone marrow depression. Bleomycin's toxicities include edema of the hands, alopecia, and stomatitis. Cisplatin produces both nephrotoxicity and ototoxicity. The clinical toxicity of vincristine is mostly neurologic. Doxorubicin causes cardiotoxicity as well as alopecia and bone marrow depression. The cardiotoxicity has been linked to a lipid peroxidation within cardiac cells.

125. The answer is C. *(AMA Drug Evaluations Annual, 1994, p 1990. DiPalma, 4/e, p 656. Gilman, 8/e, pp 1223–1224.)* Antimetabolites of folic acids such as methotrexate, which is an important cancer chemotherapeutic agent, exert their effect by inhibiting the catalytic activity of the enzyme dihydrofolate reductase. The enzyme functions to keep folic acid in a reduced state. The first step in the reaction is the reduction of folic acid to 7,8-dihydrofolic acid (FH_2), which requires the cofactor NADPH. The second step is the conversion of 7,8-dihydrofolic acid to 5,6,7,8-tetrahydrofolic acid (FH_4). This part of the reduction reaction requires NADH or NADPH. The reduced forms of folic acid are involved in one-carbon transfer reactions that are required during the synthesis of purines and pyrimidine thymidylate. The affinity of methotrexate for dihydrofolate reductase is much greater than for the substrates of folic acid and dihydrofolic acid. The action of methotrexate can be blocked or reduced by the administration of leucovorin (N^5-formyl FH_4), which can substitute for the reduced forms of folic acid in the cell. Methotrexate affects the S phase of the cell cycle. The drug is actively transported into the cell and at very large doses the drug can enter the cell by simple diffusion.

Although cladribine is an antimetabolite, it does not inhibit dihydrofolate reductase. Procarbazine, paclitaxel, and ifosfamide exert their anticancer effects through other mechanisms of action that are not associated with dihydrofolate reductase.

126. The answer is A. *(DiPalma, 4/e, p 671. Gilman, 8/e, pp 1208, 1237.)* The vinca alkaloids vincristine and vinblastine have proved valuable because they work on a different principle from most cancer chemotherapeutic agents. They (like colchicine) inhibit mitosis in metaphase by their ability to bind to tubulin. This prevents the formation of tubules and consequently the orderly arrangement of chromosomes, which apparently causes cell death.

127. The answer is D. *(DiPalma, 4/e, pp 653–656. Gilman, 8/e, pp 1202–1207.)* "Cell cycle–specific" cytotoxic agents are most effective in malignancies in which a large portion of the population of malignant cells is undergoing mitosis. In leukemia, lymphoma, choriocarcinoma, and other rapidly growing tumors, these agents may induce a high-percentage cell kill of the entire tumor and at least of those cells that are actively dividing. In slowly growing, solid tumors, such as carcinomas of the colon, the frequency of actively dividing cells is low, and perhaps the resting cells survive the cycle-specific agents and then can be recruited back into the proliferative cycle.

128. The answer is D. *(AMA Drug Evaluations Annual, 1993, pp 1174–1175. DiPalma, 4/e, pp 668–669.)* The potential serious adverse effect of bleomycin is pneumonitis and pulmonary fibrosis. This adverse effect appears to be both age- and dose-related. The clinical onset is characterized by decreasing pulmonary function, fine rales, cough, and diffuse basilar infiltrates. This complication develops in approximately 5 to 10 percent of patients treated with bleomycin. Thus, extreme caution must be used in patients with a preexisting history of pulmonary disease. All the other drugs listed in the question are effective against carcinomas and have not been associated with significant lung toxicity.

129. The answer is D. *(DiPalma, 4/e, pp 654–656. Gilman, 8/e, p 1220.)* Cell cycle–specific agents such as mercaptopurine, fluorouracil, bleomycin, and vincristine have proved to be the most effective against proliferating cells. Busulfan is an alkylating agent that binds to DNA and causes damage to these macromolecules. It is useful against low-growth as well as high-growth tumors and is classified as a cell cycle–nonspecific agent.

130. The answer is C. *(DiPalma, 4/e, pp 653–656. Katzung, 6/e, pp 823–826.)* Cancer chemotherapy, even with the best and most efficient detection procedures, can cure only approximately 50 percent of all newly diagnosed cancer patients. The reason for failure to cure is not delay in diagnosis. Surgery, chemotherapy, and radiation constitute the three forms of treatment for cancer, but only chemotherapy can effectively treat systemic disease. Both normal and cancerous dividing cells are killed by chemotherapy, which is one of its major drawbacks. Other serious side effects include nausea, vomiting, and suppression of bone marrow. The newer agents are specifically designed for their specific effects on the cell cycle.

131. The answer is E. *(DiPalma, 4/e, pp 672–673. Gilman, 8/e, p 1256.)* Paclitaxel is a large structural molecule that contains a 15-membered taxane ring system. This anticancer agent is derived from the bark of the Pacific yew tree. Its chemotherapeutic action is related to the microtubules in the cell. Paclitaxel promotes microtubule assembly from dimers and causes microtubule stabilization by preventing depolymerization. As a consequence of these actions, the microtubules form disorganized bundles, which decreases interphase and mitotic function. Furthermore, paclitaxel also causes premature cell division. The drug is administered intravenously and is useful in such diseases as cisplatin-resistant ovarian cancer, metastatic breast cancer, malignant melanoma, and acute myelogenous leukemia. Adverse reactions reported from the use of paclitaxel include dose-dependent neutropenia, hypersensitivity reactions, mild neuropathy, transient myalgias and arthralgias, and rarely bradyarrhythmias. The cancer therapeutic agent that competitively inhibits the binding of estradiol to estrogen receptors is the oral antiestrogen tamoxifen, which is employed in the treatment of receptor-positive postmenopausal women with breast cancer.

132. The answer is B. *(DiPalma, 4/e, pp 663–664. Gilman, 8/e, pp 1213–1214.)* The alkylating agents are highly reactive compounds with the ability to form covalent bonds with nucleophilic sites on molecules such as nucleic acids. This is usually accomplished through the formation of a positively charged carbonium ion. The cytotoxic effects of these agents most likely reflect their ability to bind to the nucleotides of DNA. The alkylators have an effect during any part of the cell cycle (cell cycle–nonspecific). Because of their nonspecificity, these compounds produce a significant number of adverse effects in the host.

133. The answer is E. *(DiPalma, 4/e, pp 659–660.)* Allopurinol is a very effective inhibitor of the enzyme that metabolizes xanthine and hypoxanthine to form uric acid. This enzyme, xanthine oxidase, also is responsible for the oxidation of 6-mercaptopurine. Allopurinol, by blocking this reaction, increases the exposure time of tumor cells to 6-mercaptopurine. In addition, through the same mechanism the production of uric acid will decrease in the serum but there is no increase in uric acid levels in the urine.

134. The answer is D. *(DiPalma, 4/e, pp 681–683. Gilman, 8/e, pp 1267–1270.)* Cyclosporine is not cytotoxic in the ordinary sense and hence does not depress bone marrow. This makes it suitable for immunosuppression in bone marrow transplants. Despite its large molecular size it crosses cell membranes easily and binds to a cytoplasmic protein known as cyclophilin. It selectively inhibits the activation of T cells. The production of IL-2 is greatly reduced by the action of cyclosporine on helper T cells. The ring structure of cyclosporine is resistant to cell attack, but the side chains are oxidized by the cytochrome P-450 liver enzyme system. Excretion is mainly via the bile and little cyclosporine appears in the urine.

135. The answer is C. *(DiPalma, 4/e, pp 677, 679–680. Gilman, 8/e, pp 1270–1271.)* Azathioprine is converted in the body to mercaptopurine. It is well absorbed in the GI tract and this is the main avenue of administration. As a cytotoxic drug it suppresses all cells and especially rapidly growing ones. Thus the bone marrow and the GI mucosa are growth-inhibited. This gives rise to the GI symptoms and the increased incidence of infections. Late toxicity includes the increased risk of malignancy, especially skin cancers and lymphoid tumors.

136. The answer is E. *(AMA Drug Evaluations Annual, 1993, p 2000. DiPalma, 4/e, pp 657, 659–660.)* Fludarabine phosphate is classified as a purine derivative with antineoplastic properties. The drug is rapidly dephosphorylated in plasma. A carrier-mediated transport system takes fludarabine into the cell, where it is phosphorylated to a triphosphate compound. It is the triphosphate form of the drug that inhibits DNA polymerase following its incorporation in DNA. Fludarabine also is cytotoxic in nondividing cells through the inhibition of DNA ligase I. The drug has been used in the treatment of chlorambucil-resistant chronic lymphocytic leukemia, myeloid leukemia, and indolent non-Hodgkin's lymphoma. The primary toxicity associated with fludarabine is reversible myelosuppression. Some other adverse reactions that are attributed to this purine derivative are peripheral sensorimotor neuropathy and neurologic symptoms, such as cortical blindness, optic neuritis, and seizures. Fludarabine is biotransformed by dephosphorylation. The enzyme xanthine oxidase is involved in the biotransformation of the purine derivative mercaptopurine. Since mercaptopurine is degraded by xanthine oxidase, allopurinol, which is a xanthine oxidase inhibitor, must be used with caution in the presence of mercaptopurine because allopurinol can increase the toxicities of mercaptopurine.

137. The answer is A. *(DiPalma, 4/e, pp 643, 678–679. Gilman, 8/e, pp 1443–1445.)* Glucocorticoids do not significantly diminish the concentration of antibodies in the circulation. Rather their action concerns the B- and T-cell function of producing immune substances and leukotrienes. Their anti-inflammatory actions are probably related to the inhibition of the synthesis of prostaglandins. As sole agents they are not capable of preventing graft rejection but they are useful in conjunction with azathioprine and cyclosporine.

138. The answer is D. *(DiPalma, 4/e, pp 308, 681–683. Gilman, 8/e, pp 1267–1270.)* Cyclosporine is an immunosuppressive drug classified as a specific T-cell inhibitor. The compound was isolated from a fungus and consists of 11 amino acids arranged in a cyclic structure. Although it is a relatively large molecule, cyclosporine readily crosses cellular membranes. The drug is absorbed upon oral administration; however, the extent of absorption is approximately 30 percent of that obtained following intravenous administration. As with other immunosuppressive drugs, cyclosporine can cause serious adverse reactions. Nephrotoxicity is a problem with the use of this agent. In some cases, lowering of the dosage may reduce the renal toxicity; in other cases the drug must be terminated. Other adverse reactions can include hypertension, hirsutism, neurotoxicity, convulsions, hepatitis, and hyperplasia of the gums. The unusual reaction of gingival hyperplasia is similar to that produced by the antiepileptic drug phenytoin.

139. The answer is C. *(DiPalma, 4/e, pp 677–680, 684–687. Gilman, 8/e, p 1272.)* Muromonab-CD3 is a monoclonal antibody that interferes with T-cell function. It is classified as an immunosuppressive drug. This drug is given intravenously and is indicated in the treatment of acute allograft rejection. Generally, azathioprine and prednisone are used along with muromonab-CD3. Interferon alpha and aldesleukin (interleukin 2) are cytokines that are classified as immunostimulants. Sargramostim and filgrastim are also immunostimulants. These drugs are produced by recombinant DNA technology. Sargramostim is a human granulocyte macrophage colony stimulating factor (GM-CSF) and filgrastim is a human granulocyte colony stimulating factor (G-CSF).

140. The answer is E. *(DiPalma, 4/e, pp 678, 687. Gilman, 8/e, p 1230.)* Levamisole was used as an anthelmintic agent. It is now indicated in the therapy of advanced colon cancer in combination with 5-fluorouracil. Levamisole is classified as an immunostimulant; however, this action is dose-dependent and related to duration of administration. Its main effect may be due to enhancement of monocyte chemotaxis; however, it also causes increased monocyte phagocytosis and increased activity of neutrophils. Levamisole produces adverse reactions such as flulike symptoms, nausea, vomiting, blurred vision, convulsions, and a metallic taste. In addition, the drug may cause an alteration in the sense of smell.

141–143. The answers are 141-C, 142-D, 143-E. *(DiPalma, 4/e, pp 666–669. Gilman, 8/e, pp 1206–1207.)* Streptozocin is a nitrosourea-like antibiotic that contains a glucosamine moiety that allows it to be selectively taken up by the beta cells of the islets of Langerhans. Consequently, it appears to be useful in treating metastatic islet cell carcinoma.

Dacarbazine (DTIC) is a triazene derivative of alkylating agents that appears to require demethylation for activity. It has displayed significant antineoplastic action against malignant melanomas.

Mitomycin is a potent antibiotic that selectively inhibits DNA synthesis by its ability to alkylate and cross-link DNA. The drug causes a bone marrow suppression in up to 64 percent of patients.

144–146. The answers are 144-C, 145-F, 146-I. *(DiPalma, 4/e, pp 656–659, 661, 672, 677–681, 687–689.)* Methotrexate is classified as an antimetabolite with therapeutic uses in cancer chemotherapy and as an immunosuppressive agent indicated in the treatment of severe active classical rheumatoid arthritis. Leucovorin is related to methotrexate in that it is an antagonist of its actions. It can supply a source of reduced folate for the methylation reactions that are prevented by methotrexate.

Azathioprine is a derivative closely related to mercaptopurine. Mercaptopurine is used as a cancer chemotherapeutic agent while azathioprine is used as an imunosuppressive agent because it is more effective than mercaptopurine in this regard. Azathioprine is used in organ transplantation, particularly kidney allografts. Like mercaptopurine, azathioprine is biotransformed to inactive product by xanthine oxidase. Allopurinol, which inhibits this enzyme, can increase the therapeutic action of azathioprine and possibly its adverse reactions. The dosage of azathioprine should be decreased in the presence of allopurinol.

BCG vaccine is a nonspecific stimulant of the reticuloendothelial system. It is an attenuated strain of *Mycobacterium bovis* that appears most effective in small, localized bladder tumors. This agent is approved for intravesicular use in bladder cancer. Adverse reactions are associated with the renal system, such as problems with urination, infection, and cystitis.

147–149. The answers are 147-D, 148-H, 149-F. *(DiPalma, 4/e, pp 662, 665–668, 672–673. Gilman, 8/e, pp 1205–1207.)* Fluorouracil is a pyrimidine antagonist that has a low neurotoxicity when compared with other fluorinated derivatives; however, its major toxicities are myelosuppression and oral or gastrointestinal ulceration. Leukopenia is the most frequent clinical manifestation of the myelosuppression.

Asparaginase is an enzyme that catalyzes the hydrolysis of serum asparagine to aspartic acid and ammonia. Major toxicities are related to antigenicity and pancreatitis. In addition, more than 50 percent of those treated present biochemical evidence of hepatic dysfunction.

Procarbazine commonly produces a dose-related, reversible bone marrow depression including thrombocytopenia and leukopenia. Neurotoxicity is also associated with this drug in 10 to 20 percent of the patients receiving it. This is manifested as ataxia, disorders in consciousness, and peripheral neuropathies. Procarbazine may reduce plasma pyridoxal phosphate levels, a phenomenon that may be responsible for the neurotoxicity.

150–152. The answers are 150-B, 151-D, 152-E. *(DiPalma, 4/e, pp 653–656, 667–668.)* Specific cell-cycle events are present in both normal and cancerous cells. These phases of the cell cycle are shown in the diagram with the questions. Although general statements can be made regarding the cell-cycle phases in which certain classes of chemotherapeutic agents act, some drugs listed in a particular category of antineoplastic agents may exhibit their effects on a different phase of the cell cycle. Alkylating agents are considered to be nonspecific in regard to the phase at which they have their effects. However, the alkylating agents dacarbazine and busulfan are mostly active during the G_2 phase and the G_0 phase, respectively. In addition, antibiotic chemotherapeutic agents are considered to have effect in the G_2 phase of the cell cycle. The antibiotic agent dactinomycin, however, is most active in the S phase.

Cardiovascular and Pulmonary Systems

Cardiac Glycosides
- Digoxin, digitoxin, deslanoside

Other Inotropic Agents
- Sympathomimetics
  - Epinephrine,* isoproterenol,* dopamine,* dobutamine
- Nonsympathomimetics
  - Theophylline,* amrinone,* milrinone

Vasodilators for Congestive Heart Failure
- Nitrates, sodium nitroprusside, captopril, enalapril, lisinopril, quinapril, ramipril, nifedipine, nicardipine

Antiarrhythmic Drugs
- 1A. Quinidine,* procainamide, disopyramide
- 1B. Lidocaine,* tocainide, mexiletine, phenytoin
- 1C. Flecainide,* encainide, propafenone
- 2. Propranolol (other beta blockers)
- 3. Amiodarone,* bretylium, sotalol
- 4. Verapamil, diltiazem
- 5. Adenosine

Antianginal Drugs
- Nitrates and nitrites
  - Nitroglycerine,* amyl nitrite, pentaerythritol tetranitrate, isosorbide dinitrate
- Beta-adrenergic blocking drugs
  - (All members are useful; a good choice is the cardioselective ones such as acebutolol, atenolol, and metoprolol.)
- Calcium channel blockers
  - Nifedipine, verapamil, diltiazem, bepridil
- Agents for hyperlipoproteinemia
  - Bile acid sequestrants
  - Colestipol, cholestyramine
  - Nicotinic acid
  - Clofibrate, gemfibrozil
  - Probucol
  - Lovastatin
  - Dehydrothyroxine

Antihypertensive Drugs
- Thiazides
  - (All are effective; most commonly used are chlorothiazide and hydrochlorothiazide—see section on Diuretics)
- Sympatholytic agents
  - Centrally acting
    - Methyldopa, clonidine, guanabenz, guanfacine
  - Peripherally acting
    - Beta-adrenergic blocking agents
      - Propranolol, etc.

- Alpha-adrenergic blocking agents
  - Prazosin, terazosin, reserpine, guanethidine, guanadrel
- Arterial vasodilators
  - Hydralazine, minoxidil
- Angiotensin-converting enzyme (ACE) inhibitors
  - Captopril, enalapril, lisinopril, quinapril, fosinopril, ramipril
- Calcium channel blockers
  - Nifedipine, verapamil, diltiazem, amlodipine, nicardipine
- Drugs for hypertensive emergencies
  - Trimethaphan, sodium nitroprusside, diazoxide, nifedipine, labetalol

Drugs for Chronic Obstructive Pulmonary Diseases (COPD)

- Bronchodilators
  - Methylxanthines, theophylline, elixophyllin
  - Beta-receptor agonists
    - Epinephrine, isoproterenol, isoetharine, metaproterenol, terbutaline, albuterol
- Anticholinergics
  - Atropine, ipratropium*
  - Mediator-release inhibitors
    - Cromolyn sodium*, nedocromil
  - Corticosteroids
    - Flunisolide, beclomethasone, triamcinolone
- Mucokinetic agents
  - Acetylcysteine
  - Guaifenesin
  - Iodide
  - Saline

Hematologic Agents

- Antianemia drugs
  - Iron-ferrous sulfate, vitamin B_{12}, folic acid
  - Iron detoxifiers, deferoxamine
- Anticoagulant and procoagulant drugs
  - Parenteral anticoagulants
    - Heparin and enoxaparin
  - Oral anticoagulants
    - Warfarin and dicumarol
  - Inhibitors of platelet aggregation
    - Aspirin and NSAIDS
  - Fibrinolytic drugs
    - Streptokinase, tissue-type plasminogen activator (t-PA, alteplase), anistreplase
- Procoagulant drugs
  - Systemic
    - Antihemophilic factor, factor VIII, factor IX complex, desmopressin, aminocaproic acid, tranexamic acid
  - Topical
    - Thrombin, absorbable gelatin, oxidized cellulose

DIRECTIONS: Each question below contains five suggested responses. Select the **one best** response to each question.

153. The cardiovascular responses of a normal man were recorded and are shown in the accompanying figure following a 15-min infusion of drug X. Which of the following was most likely drug X?

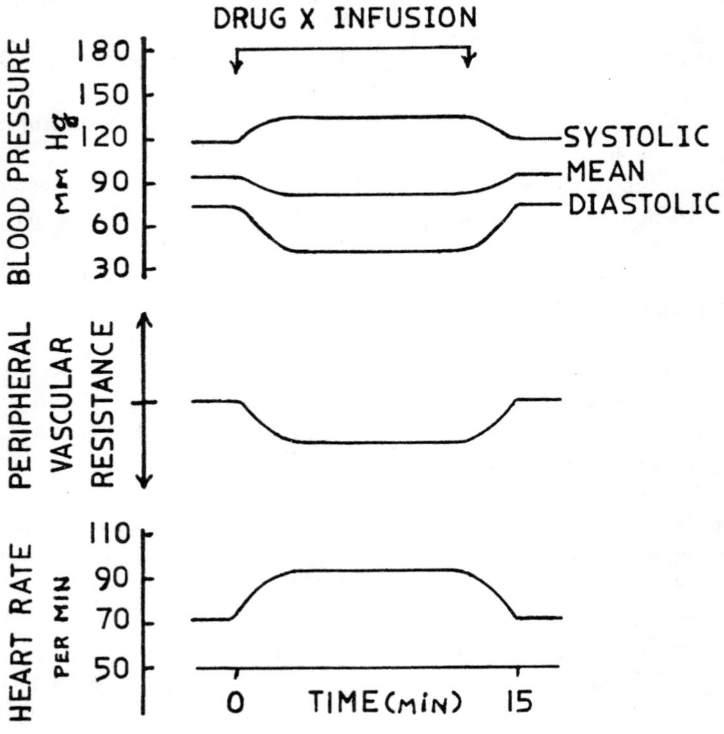

(A) Methacholine
(B) Propranolol
(C) Atropine
(D) Isoproterenol
(E) Norepinephrine

154. The drug of choice for the prevention of deep vein thrombosis following hip replacement surgery is

(A) alteplase
(B) enoxaparin
(C) desmopressin
(D) streptokinase
(E) aspirin

155. In a patient who has had attacks of paroxysmal atrial tachycardia, an ideal prophylactic drug is

(A) adenosine
(B) procainamide
(C) lidocaine
(D) nifedipine
(E) verapamil

156. The therapeutic action of beta-adrenergic receptor blockers such as propranolol in angina pectoris is believed to be primarily the result of

(A) reduced production of catecholamines
(B) dilation of the coronary vasculature
(C) decreased requirement for myocardial oxygen
(D) increased peripheral resistance
(E) increased sensitivity to catecholamines

157. Drugs that antagonize the actions of adenosine include

(A) beta blockers
(B) potassium
(C) benzodiazepine
(D) theophylline
(E) calcium channel blockers

158. A positive Coombs' test and hemolytic anemia may follow the administration of which antihypertensive drug?

(A) Methyldopa
(B) Clonidine
(C) Guanabenz
(D) Prazosin
(E) Captopril

159. Which of the following is an antiarrhythmic agent that has relatively few electrophysiologic effects on normal myocardial tissue but suppresses the arrhythmogenic tendencies of ischemic myocardial tissues?

(A) Propranolol
(B) Procainamide
(C) Quinidine
(D) Lidocaine
(E) Disopyramide

160. Inhibitors of angiotensin-converting enzyme must be used with caution in elderly persons because they are apt to cause

(A) skin rashes
(B) drug fever
(C) hepatic injury
(D) renal failure
(E) bone marrow depression

161. Cromolyn has been found to be a useful drug in chronic obstructive pulmonary disease, especially asthma. It is believed to exert a beneficial effect because it is

(A) a bronchodilator
(B) an H_1 receptor blocker
(C) an anticholinergic
(D) an inhibitor of mediator release
(E) a $beta_2$ agonist

162. Which of the following drugs recommended for the lowering of blood cholesterol inhibits the synthesis of cholesterol by blocking 3-hydroxy-3-methylglutaryl–coenzyme A (HMG-CoA) reductase?

(A) Lovastatin
(B) Probucol
(C) Clofibrate
(D) Gemfibrozil
(E) Nicotinic acid

163. The ECG of a patient who is receiving digitalis in the therapeutic dose range would be likely to show

(A) prolongation of the QT interval
(B) prolongation of the PR interval
(C) symmetric peaking of the T wave
(D) widening of the QRS complex
(E) elevation of the ST segment

164. A person is likely to be more susceptible to digoxin toxicity if digitoxin is taken with which of the following drugs?

(A) Neomycin
(B) Hydrochlorothiazide
(C) Phenobarbital
(D) Thioridazine
(E) Estradiol

165. In a hypertensive patient who is taking insulin to treat diabetes, which of the following drugs is to be used with extra caution and advice to the patient?

(A) Hydralazine
(B) Prazosin (Minipress)
(C) Guanethidine (Ismelin)
(D) Propranolol (Inderal)
(E) Methyldopa (Aldomet)

166. Which of the following drugs is considered to be most effective in relieving and preventing ischemic episodes in patients with variant angina?

(A) Propranolol
(B) Nitroglycerine
(C) Sodium nitroprusside
(D) Verapamil
(E) Isorbide dinitrate

167. The enhancement of contractility of the cardiac muscle fiber brought about by digitalis is related to

(A) increased cyclic AMP
(B) stimulation of calmodulin
(C) inhibition of the sodium pump
(D) beta-adrenergic stimulation
(E) increased production of adenosine

168. If quinidine and digoxin are administered concurrently, which of the following effects does quinidine have on digoxin?

(A) The absorption of digoxin from the GI tract is decreased
(B) The metabolism of digoxin is prevented
(C) The concentration of digoxin in the plasma is increased
(D) The effect of digoxin on the AV node is antagonized
(E) The ability of digoxin to inhibit the Na^+,K^+-stimulated ATPase is reduced

169. Drugs that block the catecholamine uptake process—such as cocaine, tricyclic antidepressants, and phenothiazines—are apt to block the antihypertensive action of which of the following drugs?

(A) Propranolol
(B) Guanethidine
(C) Prazosin
(D) Hydralazine
(E) Diazoxide

170. Which of the following causes increased synthesis and secretion of aldosterone by the adrenal cortex?

(A) Renin
(B) Angiotensin I
(C) Angiotensin II
(D) Kallikrein
(E) Kininogen

171. Which of the following antihypertensive drugs produces most of its effects by blocking $alpha_1$-adrenergic receptors in arterioles and venules?

(A) Pindolol
(B) Prazosin
(C) Minoxidil
(D) Phentolamine
(E) Clonidine

172. Nicotinic acid in the large doses used to treat hyperlipoproteinemia causes a cutaneous flush. The vasodilatory effect is due to

(A) release of histamine
(B) production of local prostaglandins
(C) release of platelet-derived growth factor (PDGF)
(D) production of nitric oxide (NO)
(E) calcium channel block

173. One type of hyperlipoproteinemia is characterized by elevated plasma levels of chylomicrons, normal plasma levels of β-lipoproteins, and the inability of any known drug to reduce lipoprotein levels. This is which of the following types of hyperlipoproteinemia?

(A) Type I
(B) Type IIa, IIb
(C) Type III
(D) Type IV
(E) Type V

174. Which of the following drugs would be indicated in a patient who still has heart failure after adequate therapy with diuretics and digoxin?

(A) Dobutamine
(B) Hydralazine
(C) Minoxidil
(D) Prazosin
(E) Enalapril

175. Angiotensin-converting enzyme (ACE) inhibitors are associated with a high incidence of which of the following adverse reactions?

(A) Hepatitis
(B) Hypokalemia
(C) Agranulocytosis
(D) Proteinuria
(E) Hirsutism

176. Digitalis is given to patients with atrial fibrillation because it

(A) decreases the excitability of the atria
(B) increases conductivity in the AV node
(C) decreases automaticity of the atria
(D) increases the effective refractory period in the AV node
(E) has muscarinic effects

177. Patients with genetically low levels of *N*-acetyltransferase are more prone to develop a lupus erythematosus–like syndrome with which of the following drugs?

(A) Propranolol (Inderal)
(B) Procainamide
(C) Digitoxin
(D) Captopril
(E) Lidocaine

178. Which of the following anemias would be treated with cyanocobalamin (vitamin B_{12})?

(A) Anemia in infants who are undergoing rapid growth
(B) Anemia associated with chelosis, dysphagia, gastritis, and hypochlorhydria
(C) Anemia associated with small, bizarre cells poorly filled with hemoglobin
(D) Anemia associated with infestation by *Diphyllobothrium latum*
(E) Bleeding from a gastric ulcer

179. The preferred agent to combat extreme digitalis overdose is

(A) potassium
(B) calcium
(C) phenytoin
(D) Fab fragments of digitalis antibodies
(E) magnesium

180. Significant relaxation of smooth muscle of both venules and arterioles is produced by which of the following drugs?

(A) Hydralazine
(B) Minoxidil (Loniten)
(C) Diazoxide (Hyperstat)
(D) Sodium nitroprusside
(E) Nifedipine

181. Precautions advisable when using lovastatin include

(A) serum transaminase measurements
(B) renal function studies
(C) acoustic measurements
(D) monthly complete blood counts
(E) avoidance of bile acid sequestrants

182. The first-line drug for treating an acute attack of reentrant supraventricular tachycardia is

(A) adenosine
(B) digitalis
(C) propranolol
(D) phenylephrine
(E) edrophonium

DIRECTIONS: Each numbered question or incomplete statement below is NEGATIVELY phrased. Select the **one best** lettered response.

183. Caffeine and other methylxanthines useful in chronic obstructive pulmonary disease (COPD) have all the following pharmacologic actions EXCEPT

(A) increased secretion of acid and pepsin by the stomach
(B) constriction of central blood vessels
(C) relaxation of bronchial smooth muscle
(D) stimulation of cyclic AMP phosphodiesterase
(E) antagonism of adenosine receptors

184. All the following drugs may be used for the therapy of life-threatening hypertensive emergency (crisis) EXCEPT

(A) furosemide
(B) diazoxide
(C) nifedipine
(D) labetalol
(E) pindolol

185. For the monotherapy of mild-to-moderate hypertension, all the following drugs would be suitable EXCEPT

(A) metoprolol
(B) minoxidil
(C) verapamil
(D) enalapril
(E) nifedipine

186. Nitroglycerine, a frequently used cardiovascular drug, has all the following actions EXCEPT

(A) it can cause adverse reactions of headache and tachycardia
(B) it undergoes significant first-pass biotransformation
(C) it is used for congestive heart failure
(D) it decreases total coronary blood flow
(E) it is converted to nitrite by the smooth muscle cell

187. True statements regarding the mechanism of action of the nitrites and organic nitrates in causing smooth muscle relaxation include all the following EXCEPT

(A) nitric oxide (NO) is formed
(B) adenyl cyclase is inhibited
(C) a cyclic GMP–dependent protein kinase is stimulated
(D) the light chain of myosin is dephosphorylated
(E) the mechanism is similar to that of endothelial-derived relaxing factor (EDRF)

188. All the following deficiencies or agents may cause megaloblastic anemia EXCEPT

(A) deficiency of folic acid
(B) methotrexate therapy for leukemia
(C) trimethoprim therapy
(D) phenytoin therapy for epilepsy
(E) L-dopa therapy of parkinsonism

189. The automaticity of Purkinje's fibers of the heart can be increased by all the following EXCEPT

(A) epinephrine
(B) digitalis
(C) quinidine
(D) low concentrations of potassium
(E) isoproterenol

190. Beta-adrenergic blocking agents have a beneficial effect in angina because they do all the following EXCEPT

(A) slow the heart rate
(B) lower blood pressure
(C) buffer the heart against sympathetic stimulation
(D) cause peripheral vasodilation
(E) reduce myocardial contractility

191. The nitrates remain the most valuable agents for the therapy of angina pectoris. Valid statements with respect to their overall mechanism of action include all the following EXCEPT

(A) nitrates cause reflex tachycardia
(B) in normal subjects nitrates can induce a transient increase in total coronary flow by directly dilating coronary arteries
(C) in coronary artery disease beneficial actions of nitrates are attributable to a decreased myocardial oxygen requirement
(D) nitrates increase venous capacitance and thus cause a decrease in myocardial preload
(E) nitrates are incompatible with beta blockers

192. Calcium channel blocking drugs have gained wide prominence in recent years. They relate to the role of calcium in the control function of several organ systems. All the following may be altered therapeutically by restricting calcium influx EXCEPT

(A) vascular smooth muscle
(B) skeletal muscle
(C) cardiac muscle
(D) glandular secretion
(E) esophageal smooth muscle

193. Drugs that reduce the size of a preformed fibrin clot have recently proved to be especially useful. Agents capable of dissolving fibrin clots include all the following EXCEPT

(A) tissue plasminogen activator (tPA)
(B) urokinase
(C) streptokinase
(D) factor IX complex
(E) anistreplase (streptokinase-plasminogen complex)

194. Megaloblastic anemia may be responsive to administration of all the following EXCEPT

(A) cyanocobalamin
(B) intrinsic factor concentrate
(C) ferrous sulfate
(D) folic acid
(E) folinic acid

195. Endogenous heparin is characterized by all the following statements EXCEPT

(A) it is found largely in mast cells
(B) it is a sulfonated mucopolysaccharide
(C) it is inhibited by protamine sulfate
(D) it is able to release a lipemia-clearing factor
(E) it crosses the placental barrier

196. Antiarrhythmic drugs used prophylactically to prevent sustained, ventricular tachycardia may be accompanied by all the following benefits and adverse reactions EXCEPT

(A) reduced number of premature ventricular contractions
(B) elimination of runs of nonsustained ventricular tachycardia
(C) torsades de pointes with class I antiarrhythmic drugs
(D) prolonged life expectancy in most cases
(E) relief of symptomatic premature ventricular contractions

197. The bipyridines amrinone and milrinone have gained acceptance as useful inotropic agents in congestive heart failure. Beneficial actions include an increase in all the following EXCEPT

(A) intracellular calcium
(B) cardiac output
(C) Na^+,K^+-ATPase activity
(D) peripheral vasodilation
(E) protein kinase activity

198. Drugs that cause bronchodilation include all the following EXCEPT

(A) theophylline
(B) albuterol
(C) ephedrine
(D) cromolyn
(E) ipratropium

DIRECTIONS: Each group of questions below consists of lettered headings followed by a set of numbered items. For each numbered item select the **one** lettered heading with which it is **most** closely associated. Each lettered heading may be used **once, more than once, or not at all.**

Questions 199–200

Listed below are drugs designed to lower blood cholesterol. For each of these drugs select the most appropriate mechanism of action.

(A) Inhibits lipolysis in adipose tissue
(B) Decreases cholesterol synthesis at a rate-limiting step
(C) Increases the excretion of bile acids
(D) Decreases esterification of triglycerides in the liver and increases the activity of lipoprotein lipase
(E) Increases the activity of the lipid-clearing factor of heparin

199. Cholestyramine (Questran)

200. Nicotinic acid

Questions 201–202

Match the major mechanism of action with the appropriate antihypertensive drug.

(A) Guanfacine
(B) Prazosin
(C) Minoxidil
(D) Propranolol
(E) Captopril
(F) Diltiazem

201. Stimulation of $alpha_2$-adrenergic receptors in the nucleus tractus solitarius

202. Selective blocking of peripheral postsynaptic $alpha_1$-adrenergic receptors

Questions 203–205

Match each route of administration and treatment indication with the correct drug.

(A) Isoproterenol
(B) Terbutaline
(C) Nitroglycerine
(D) Cromolyn sodium
(E) Beclomethasone
(F) Sodium nitroprusside

203. Administered transdermally for angina pectoris

204. Administered parenterally to produce myocardial stimulation

205. Administered by aerosol for bronchial asthma

Questions 206–207

The calcium channel blockers have proved useful in a number of cardiovascular conditions. Match the following qualifications to the appropriate drug.

(A) Amlodipine
(B) Bepridil
(C) Diltiazem
(D) Nifedipine
(E) Verapamil

206. FDA approval for vasospastic angina, chronic stable angina, atrial flutter and fibrillation, paroxysmal atrial tachycardia, and essential hypertension

207. Most ability to reduce peripheral vascular resistance without slowing of the AV nodal conduction or reduction of cardiac contractility

Questions 208–209

It is customary today to classify antiarrhythmic drugs according to their mechanism of action. This is best defined by intracellular recordings that yield monophasic action potentials. In the accompanying figure, the monophasic action potentials of (A) slow response fiber (SA node) and (B) fast Purkinje fiber are shown. For each description that follows, choose the appropriate drug with which the change in character of the monophasic action potential is likely to be associated.

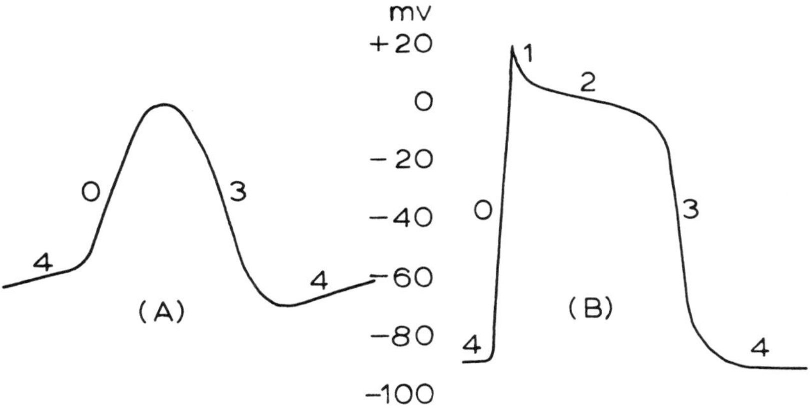

(A) Digitalis
(B) Amiodarone (Cordarone)
(C) Mexiletine (Mexitil)
(D) Nifedipine (Procardia)
(E) Propranolol (Inderal)
(F) Flecainide (Tambocor)
(G) Disopyramide (Norpace)
(H) Verapamil (Calan, Isoptin)

208. Moderate phase 0 depression and slow conduction; prolonged repolarization

209. Affects mainly phase 3, prolonging repolarization

Questions 210–212

Match the mechanism of preventing or relieving bronchospasm with the correct drug.

(A) Corticosteroids
(B) Cromolyn
(C) Theophylline
(D) Albuterol
(E) Acetylcysteine
(F) Ipratropium

210. Prevents reflex stimulation of upper and lower airways, esophagus, and carotid bodies

211. Breaks down sputum molecules to smaller components

212. Inhibits mediator release from inflammatory cells

Questions 213–215

Match the drugs below with the appropriate action.

(A) Raises the plasma level of factor IX
(B) Inhibits thrombin and early coagulation steps
(C) Inhibits synthesis of prothrombin
(D) Inhibits platelet aggregation in vitro
(E) Activates plasminogen
(F) Binds the calcium ion cofactor in some coagulation steps

213. Coumarin derivatives

214. Dipyridamole

215. Ethylenediaminetetraacetic acid (EDTA)

Questions 216–217

Match each anemia with the agent to which it best responds.

(A) Ferrous sulfate
(B) Vitamin B_{12}
(C) Folic acid
(D) Intrinsic factor
(E) Erythropoietin
(F) Copper
(G) Ascorbic acid

216. Anemia associated with advanced renal disease that requires dialysis

217. Macrocytic anemia associated with chronic alcoholism

Questions 218–220

Match the descriptions below with the appropriate agent.

(A) Angiotensin I
(B) Angiotensin II
(C) Clonidine
(D) Saralasin
(E) Captopril

218. Formed by sequential enzymatic cleavage by renin and then peptidyl dipeptidase (kinase II)

219. An octapeptide that lowers blood pressure in renin-dependent hypertensive patients

220. Lowers blood pressure in hypertensive patients by inhibiting peptidyl dipeptidase

Questions 221–222

The available drugs for promoting coagulation have diverse mechanisms of action. Match the mechanisms with the appropriate drug.

(A) Antihemophilic factor
(B) Desmopressin
(C) Factor IX complex
(D) Aminocaproic acid
(E) Oxidized cellulose

221. Increases the titers of endogenous clotting factors

222. Inhibits the fibrinolytic mechanism

Cardiovascular and Pulmonary Systems

Answers

153. The answer is D. *(DiPalma, 4/e, pp 116–122, 133–134. Gilman, 8/e, pp 192–202.)* Only isoproterenol will lower mean blood pressure, decrease peripheral vascular resistance, and increase heart rate. Methacholine decreases heart rate as does propranolol. Atropine has no action on peripheral resistance. Norepinephrine causes intense vasoconstriction and raises the mean blood pressure.

154. The answer is B. *(DiPalma, 4/e, pp 528, 533–535. Isselbacher, 13/e, pp 1140–1142.)* Deep vein thrombosis may be prevented by anticoagulants. Heparin and oral anticoagulants such as warfarin are often used. Enoxaparin is a low-molecular-weight heparin with the advantage of greater duration of action. Remarkably it seems to work without altering laboratory values of coagulation factors. Aspirin is sometimes used in conjunction with antithrombolytic agents, but alone it would be ineffective. Streptokinase can only be given once and alteplase is extremely expensive. Desmopressin is a procoagulant drug and would be contraindicated.

155. The answer is E. *(DiPalma, 4/e, pp 421–423. Gilman, 8/e, pp 624–625, 869–870.)* Because verapamil, a calcium channel blocker, has a selective depressing action on AV nodal tissue, it is an ideal drug for both immediate and prophylactic therapy of supraventricular tachycardia. Nifedipine, another calcium channel blocker, has little effect on supraventricular arrhythmia. Lidocaine and adenosine are parenteral drugs with short half-lives and thus are not suitable for prophylactic therapy. Procainamide is more suitable for ventricular arrhythmias and has the potential for serious adverse reactions with long-term use.

156. The answer is C. *(DiPalma, 4/e, pp 429–430. Gilman, 8/e, p 780.)* Beta-adrenergic receptor blockers cause a slowing of heart rate, lower blood pressure, and lessened cardiac contractility without reducing cardiac output. There is also a buffering action against adrenergic stimulation of the cardiac autoregulatory mechanism. These hemodynamic actions decrease the requirement of the heart for oxygen.

157. The answer is D. *(DiPalma, 4/e, p 492. Gilman, 8/e, p 624.)* Adenosine receptors (also called P_1, or purinergic, receptors) are blocked by methylxanthines such as theophylline. Adenosine is a powerful bronchoconstrictor, and it may be that theophylline exerts its beneficial action in asthma by blocking adenosine. None of the other drugs directly antagonize adenosine, although they may have indirect modulating actions.

158. The answer is A. *(DiPalma, 4/e, p 472. Isselbacher, 13/e, pp 1749–1750.)* Many drugs can cause an immunohemolytic anemia. Methyldopa may cause a positive Coombs' test in as many as 20 percent of patients along with hemolytic anemia. Other drugs with similar actions on red blood cells are penicillins, quinidine, procainamide, and sulfonamides. These form a stable or unstable hapten on the red cell surface, which induces an immune reaction (IgG antibodies) and leads to dissolution of the membrane.

159. The answer is D. *(DiPalma, 4/e, p 415. Gilman, 8/e, p 858.)* Lidocaine usually shortens the duration of the action potential and thus allows more time for recovery during diastole. It also blocks both activated and inactivated sodium channels. This has the effect of minimizing the action of lidocaine on normal myocardial tissues as contrasted to depolarized ischemic tissues. Thus lidocaine is particularly suitable for arrhythmias arising during ischemic episodes such as myocardial infarction.

160. The answer is D. *(DiPalma, 4/e, p 48. Gilman, 8/e, p 759.)* Elderly people are apt to have low-reserve kidneys owing to renal artery stenosis. Inhibitors of angiotensin-converting enzyme depress renal function and cause proteinuria even in patients with normal kidneys. In the elderly this toxicity is more manifest and may precipitate acute renal failure. The other toxicities listed in the question do not occur at a higher frequency in the elderly.

161. The answer is D. *(DiPalma, 4/e, pp 489–490. Gilman, 8/e, p 630.)* Cromolyn inhibits the release of mediators from mast cells, including histamine and slow-reacting substance of anaphylaxis (SRS-A). This prevents allergically induced bronchospasm. Cromolyn is of no use in an acute asthmatic attack but is of considerable help in prophylaxis of asthmatic attacks, particularly in children.

162. The answer is A. *(DiPalma, 4/e, p 450. Gilman, 8/e, pp 881–884.)* Lovastatin decreases cholesterol synthesis in the liver by inhibiting HMG-CoA reductase, the rate-limiting enzyme in the synthetic pathway. This results in an increase in LDL receptors in the liver, thus reducing blood levels for cholesterol. The intake of dietary cholesterol must not be increased, as this would allow the liver to use more exogenous cholesterol and defeat the action of lovastatin.

163. The answer is B. *(DiPalma, 4/e, p 391. Gilman, 8/e, p 824.)* The usual electrocardiographic pattern of a patient receiving therapeutic doses of digitalis includes an increase in the PR interval, depression and sagging of the ST segment, and occasional biphasia or inversion of the T wave. Symmetrically peaked T waves are associated with hyperkalemia or ischemia in most cases. Shortening of the QT interval, rather than prolongation, is characteristic of digitalis treatment.

164. The answer is B. *(DiPalma, 4/e, p 356. Gilman, 8/e, p 835.)* Low body stores of potassium increase susceptibility to digitalis toxicity. The thiazide diuretics, such as hydrochlorothiazide, promote excretion of potassium. Diuretics are often given with digoxin to treat congestive heart failure; this combination frequently causes digitalis toxicity.

165. The answer is D. *(DiPalma, 4/e, p 136. Gilman, 8/e, p 239.)* Propranolol as well as other nonselective beta blockers tends to slow the rate of recovery in a hypoglycemic attack caused by insulin. Beta blockers also mask the symptoms of hypoglycemia and may actually cause hypertension because of the increased plasma epinephrine in the presence of vascular $beta_2$ blockade.

166. The answer is D. *(DiPalma, 4/e, pp 434–435. Gilman, 8/e, p 779.)* Calcium channel blockers, of which nifedipine is a prime example, are now considered to be more effective than nitrates in relieving variant angina. This is because this type of angina is believed to be caused by vasospasm, which is best antagonized by slow channel calcium blockers. Such blockers appear to have a relative selectivity for coronary arteries.

167. The answer is C. *(DiPalma, 4/e, p 390. Gilman, 8/e, p 817.)* Digitalis inhibits Na^+,K^+-stimulated ATPase and hence decreases the pumping of sodium out of the myocyte. As a result, there is a relative reduction of expulsion of calcium from the cell's sodium-calcium exchange. The consequent increased free calcium in the cell causes increased intensity of interaction between actin and myosin filaments and enhanced contractility.

168. The answer is C. *(DiPalma, 4/e, p 395. Gilman, 8/e, p 836.)* Quinidine is often given in conjunction with digitalis. It has been found by pharmacokinetic studies that this combination results in quinidine's replacing digitalis in tissue binding sites (mainly muscle), thus raising the blood level of digitalis and decreasing its volume of distribution. A mechanism by which quinidine interferes with the renal excretion of digitalis has also been proposed.

169. The answer is B. *(DiPalma, 4/e, p 144. Gilman, 8/e, p 794.)* Neuronal uptake is necessary for the hypotensive action of guanethidine. It competes for the norepinephrine storage site and in time replaces the natural neurotransmitter. This is the basis of its hypotensive effect. Drugs that prevent reuptake by the neurons, such as cocaine, would destroy the effectiveness of guanethidine.

170. The answer is C. *(DiPalma, 4/e, p 388. Gilman, 8/e, p 753.)* Angiotensin II by a direct mechanism acts on the zona glomerulosa to cause increased conversion of cholesterol to pregnenolone, which results in a greater yield of aldosterone. Angiotensin I is the precursor of angiotensin II. Renin catalyzes the conversion of angiotensin I from angiotensinogen. Kallikreins convert prorenin to active renin. Kininogens are precursors of kinins.

171. The answer is B. *(DiPalma, 4/e, pp 143, 475. Gilman, 8/e, p 226.)* Prazosin and its close relative terazosin block mainly $alpha_1$ receptors in contrast to phentolamine, which blocks both $alpha_1$ and $alpha_2$ receptors. The $alpha_1$-receptor selectivity permits the normal norepinephrine negative feedback on $alpha_2$ presynaptic receptors. Pindolol is a beta blocker; minoxidil is a direct-acting vasodilator.

172. The answer is B. *(DiPalma, 4/e, p 447. Gilman, 8/e, p 893.)* Nicotinic acid in large doses stimulates the production of prostaglandins as shown by an increase in blood level. The flush may be prevented by the prior administration of aspirin, which is known to block synthesis of prostaglandins.

173. The answer is A. *(DiPalma, 4/e, pp 444–445. Gilman, 8/e, p 881.)* In type I hyperlipoproteinemia, drugs that reduce levels of lipoproteins are not useful, but reduction of dietary sources of fat may help. Cholesterol levels are usually normal but triglycerides are elevated. Maintenance of ideal body weight is recommended in all types of hyperlipidemia. Clofibrate (Atromid-S) effectively reduces the levels of very low-density lipoproteins characteristic of types III, IV, and V hyperlipoproteinemias; and administration of cholestyramine resin and lovastatin in conjunction with a low-cholesterol diet is regarded as effective therapy for type IIa, or primary, hyperbetalipoproteinemia, except in the homozygous familial form.

174. The answer is E. *(DiPalma, 4/e, pp 397–398. Gilman, 8/e, p 758.)* Vasodilator therapy of heart failure has gained prominence in the past 10 years. The angiotensin-converting enzyme (ACE) inhibitors (enalapril) are among the best for this purpose, although calcium channel inhibitors and nitroglycerine can also be used. The ACE inhibitors dilate arterioles (reducing preload), dilate veins (reducing preload), and inhibit the production of aldosterone (reducing blood volume)—all factors considered beneficial in the therapy of congestive heart failure.

175. The answer is D. *(DiPalma, 4/e, p 481. Gilman, 8/e, p 759.)* The most consistent of the toxicities of inhibitors of angiotensin-converting enzymes is impairment of renal function evidenced by proteinuria. Elevations of BUN and creatinine occur frequently, especially when stenosis of the renal artery or severe heart failure exists. Hyperkalemia also may occur. These drugs are to be used very cautiously where prior renal failure is present and in the elderly. Other toxicities include neutropenia and angioedema. Hepatic toxicity has not been reported.

176. The answer is D. *(DiPalma, 4/e, p 394. Gilman, 8/e, pp 824–827.)* Digitalis is used in atrial fibrillation to slow the ventricular rate; the atrial fibrillation itself is not usually controlled. Digitalis acts to slow the speed of conduction and to increase the effective refractory period in the AV node, which prevents transmission of all the impulses from the atria to the ventricles. The drug exerts these effects on the AV node by direct action on the heart and by indirectly increasing vagal activity.

177. The answer is B. *(DiPalma, 4/e, pp 413–414. Gilman, 8/e, pp 856, 857.)* Persons with low hepatic *N*-acetyltransferase activity are known as slow acetylators. A major pathway of metabolism of procainamide, which is used to treat arrhythmias, is *N*-acetylation. Slow acetylators receiving this drug are more susceptible than normal persons to side effects, since slow acetylators will have higher-than-normal blood levels of these drugs. *N*-Acetylprocainamide, the metabolite of procainamide, is also active and is being tested as an antiarrhythmic agent.

178. The answer is D. *(DiPalma, 4/e, pp 507, 516. Gilman, 8/e, p 1299.)* Iron deficiency anemia usually occurs in infants undergoing rapid growth. In adults in a late stage it may result in a bowel syndrome associated with gastritis and hypochlorhydria (Plummer-Vinson syndrome). Characteristically all iron deficiency anemias are associated with a hypochromic microcytic blood profile. Infestation with the tapeworm *Diphyllobothrium latum* is accompanied by a hyperchromic macrocytic anemia treatable with vitamin B_{12}. Bleeding syndromes are treated with iron.

179. The answer is D. *(DiPalma, 4/e, p 396. Gilman, 8/e, pp 835–836.)* In digitalis overdose only the administration of a specific Fab fragment that acts as an antibody for digitalis is effective. This raises the blood level of the digitalis glycoside but it is not available for action on the heart and indeed the combined Fab fragment–digitalis complex is excreted by the kidney. While potassium, magnesium, and phenytoin will counteract some of the arrhythmogenic actions of digitalis, they are not effective in severe digitalis overdose. Calcium would augment the toxicity of digitalis.

180. The answer is D. *(DiPalma, 4/e, pp 397–398. Gilman, 8/e, p 803.)* Hydralazine, minoxidil, diazoxide, and sodium nitroprusside are all directly acting vasodilators used to treat hypertension. Because hydralazine, minoxidil, nifedipine, and diazoxide relax arteriolar smooth muscle more than smooth muscle in venules, the effect on venous capacitance is negligible. Sodium nitroprusside, which affects both arterioles and venules, does not increase cardiac output, a feature that enhances the utility of sodium nitroprusside in the management of hypertensive crisis associated with myocardial infarction.

181. The answer is A. *(DiPalma, 4/e, pp 450–452. Gilman, 8/e, pp 881–885.)* Lovastatin should not be used in patients with severe liver disease. With routine use of lovastatin, serum transaminase values may rise, and in such patients the drug may be continued only with great caution. Lovastatin has also been associated with lenticular opacities, and slit-lamp studies should be done before and 1 year after the start of therapy. There is no effect on the otic nerve. The drug is not toxic to the renal system and reports of bone marrow depression are very rare. There is a small incidence of myopathy, and levels of creatinine kinase should be measured when unexplained muscle pain occurs. Combination with cyclosporine or clofibrate has led to myopathy. There is no danger in use with bile acid sequestrants.

182. The answer is A. *(DiPalma, 4/e, pp 421–423. Isselbacher, 13/e, pp 1026–1027, 1032.)* Older therapies—all designed to favor parasympathetic control of rhythm—include digitalis, propranolol, edrophonium, and vasoconstrictors. The vasoconstrictor phenylephrine (given by intravenous bolus) causes stimulation of the carotid sinus and reflex vagal stimulation of the atria. More recently, adenosine has been favored over verapamil, which is also very effective but slower acting.

183. The answer is D. *(DiPalma, 4/e, p 492. Gilman, 8/e, pp 619–620.)* The most likely mechanism of methylxanthine action is by inhibition, not stimulation, of phosphodiesterase. This leads to an increase in cytosolic cyclic AMP and subsequent relaxation of smooth muscle. Methylxanthines also antagonize adenosine receptors. Since adenosine causes bronchoconstriction, this antagonism may also contribute to the bronchodilating action.

184. The answer is E. *(DiPalma, 4/e, pp 483–484. Gilman, 8/e, p 810.)* Beta blockers are not dilators of peripheral arterioles and lower blood pressure mainly by a negative inotropic effect on the heart. Pindolol, especially, would not be indicated for life-threatening hypertension since it also has beta$_1$-agonist properties. Labetalol is an exception since it has considerable alpha-adrenergic blocking properties in addition to being a beta blocker. Nifedipine is especially useful even by the oral route, as is furosemide, the latter by decreasing blood volume. Diazoxide, although related to thiazide diuretics, does not cause diuresis but is an effective peripheral vasodilator.

185. The answer is B. *(DiPalma, 4/e, p 477. Gilman, 8/e, p 801.)* Because long-term therapy with diuretics has led to complications of hyperkalemia, uricemia, and hypercholesterolemia, the present approach is to use monotherapy with drugs free of these side effects. Beta blockers (metoprolol), inhibitors of angiotensin-converting enzyme (enalapril), and calcium channel blockers (verapamil, nifedipine) are suitable for this purpose. Minoxidil, a direct-acting vasodilator, is indicated in multiple drug therapy in severe hypertension.

186. The answer is D. *(DiPalma, 4/e, pp 425–428. Gilman, 8/e, pp 765–769.)* Nitroglycerine is the most frequently administered antianginal drug. Its main adverse effects are headache and tachycardia in many patients. By the oral route it undergoes very active first-pass biotransformation and thus is very short-acting. Recently, it has been frequently employed in congestive heart failure because of its property of dilating the venous bed. Despite the fact that nitrates do dilate coronary vessels, most studies show that total coronary flow is not increased (it certainly is not decreased). The sulfhydril group in myocyte membranes converts nitrate to nitrite.

187. The answer is B. *(DiPalma, 4/e, pp 427–428. Gilman, 8/e, p 768.)* Adenyl cyclase is not involved. The receptor for nitrite converts NO_2 to NO. This free radical reacts with guanylate cyclase to cause increased synthesis of guanosine 3′-5′-monophosphate (cyclic GMP). A GMP-dependent protein kinase is activated; this results in decreased phosphorylation of muscle protein, which decreases muscle's capacity to contract. In this manner, nitrates relax all smooth muscles. This action of nitrites is identical to that of EDRF.

188. The answer is E. *(DiPalma, 4/e, pp 308, 511, 513, 739. Gilman, 8/e, pp 441, 1054, 1223, 1244.)* Although the cause of pernicious anemia is a deficiency of vitamin B_{12}, deficiency of folic acid may cause a similar syndrome of megaloblastic anemia. In the therapy of cancer, methotrexate—a folate analogue—causes folate deficiency and hence megaloblastic anemia. Trimethoprim is also an antifolate substance used in the chemotherapy of malaria and other bacterial infections. Ordinarily it is quite safe because its affinity for bactericidal folate reductase is greater than for that of the host; however, in large doses it can cause folate deficiency. Phenytoin, a drug widely used to treat epilepsy, can in long-term use bring about folate deficiency possibly by decreasing absorption from the gastrointestinal tract. L-Dopa therapy of Parkinson's disease does not cause megaloblastic anemia.

189. The answer is C. *(DiPalma, 4/e, pp 119, 405, 410. Gilman, 8/e, pp 195, 818–820.)* Automaticity of Purkinje's fibers is increased by epinephrine, digitalis, isoproterenol, and low concentration of potassium. It is decreased by quinidine or high concentration of potassium. The modification of automaticity is important: in complete heart block, a condition of rhythm failure with bradycardia, isoproterenol or epinephrine might be used to enhance the automaticity of the ventricular conductive system. However, in the situation of supraventricular and ventricular ectopy, all agents able to facilitate automaticity should be avoided.

190. The answer is D. *(DiPalma, 4/e, pp 429–430. Gilman, 8/e, p 780.)* Beta-adrenergic blocking agents do not cause peripheral vasodilation. The lowering of blood pressure is due to a decrease in myocardial contractility. The slowing of heart rate improves the efficiency of the heart, while the buffering effect against sympathetic stimulation prevents sudden increases in oxygen demand. The end result is a heart with a reduced oxygen requirement for a given level of work.

191. The answer is E. *(DiPalma, 4/e, pp 425–427. Gilman, 8/e, pp 765–768.)* There is no doubt that, experimentally, nitrates dilate coronary vessels. This also occurs in normal subjects, resulting in an overall increase in coronary blood flow. In arteriosclerotic coronaries, the ability to dilate is lost and the ischemic area may actually have less blood flow under the influence of nitrates. Improvement in the ischemic condition is the result of decreased myocardial oxygen demands because of a reduction of preload and afterload. Nitrates dilate both arteries and veins and thus reduce the work of the heart. As the blood pressure falls, there is reflex tachycardia. Nitrates are compatible with beta blockers, which slow the heart and counteract the reflex tachycardia caused by nitrates.

192. The answer is B. *(DiPalma, 4/e, pp 430–434. Gilman, 8/e, pp 774–778.)* Smooth muscle, especially of vasculature, depends on transmembrane calcium influx for normal resting tone and contractile responses. In contrast, skeletal muscle uses intracellular pools of calcium and does not depend on calcium influx. Cardiac muscle requires calcium influx for excitation-contraction coupling. A reduction in mechanical function of the myocardium reduces the oxygen requirement in angina pectoris. Calcium influx is required for the release of several hormones, for example insulin. However, the doses required are too large to be used routinely in humans. Esophageal spasm may be combated by nifedipine.

193. The answer is D. *(DiPalma, 4/e, pp 525, 533–534. Gilman, 8/e, p 1323. Katzung, 4/e, p 412.)* Tissue plasminogen activator, urokinase, and streptokinase, although obtained from different sources, all are capable of dissolving a fibrin clot. Tissue plasminogen activator is manufactured by a recombinant technique and is extremely expensive. It may have the advantage of causing less cerebral bleeding as compared with streptokinase and urokinase. Factor IX complex is a dried human plasma fraction that is used to promote clotting when a bleeding episode caused by a genetic acquired deficiency of these factors is evident. A combination of streptokinase and lys-plasminogen, anistreplase, has been recently introduced and may have advantages over tissue plasminogen activator or streptokinase used alone.

194. The answer is C. *(DiPalma, 4/e, pp 505–507, 511. Gilman, 8/e, pp 1294–1306.)* Vitamin B_{12} deficiency has several causes. Pernicious anemia, associated with gastric mucosal atrophy and histamine-refractory achlorhydria, eliminates the production of intrinsic factor that would combine with cyanocobalamin (B_{12}) in the gut. Parenteral administration of B_{12} is recommended for patients who have pernicious anemia. Oral B_{12} and intrinsic factor concentrate should be used only in patients who have a proven intrinsic factor deficit and refuse intramuscular administration of B_{12}. Other causes of vitamin B_{12} deficiency, in the face of normal intrinsic factor secretion, include malabsorption syndromes and parasitic competition. Alcohol-associated megaloblastic anemia is usually caused by a deficiency of folic acid. Folinic acid is used to circumvent the effects of inhibitors of dehydrofolate reductase such as methotrexate.

195. The answer is E. *(DiPalma, 4/e, pp 526–528. Gilman, 8/e, p 1313.)* Heparin, a naturally occurring anticoagulant, is localized largely in mast cells. A mucopolysaccharide, it is composed of sulfated glucosamine and glucuronic acid. Its primary action is as an antithrombin factor, for which it requires a plasma cofactor. Organic bases (protamine) are believed to inhibit heparin by neutralizing its electronegative charge. Heparin is thought to release and stabilize a lipemia-clearing factor that catalyzes the hydrolysis of triglycerides. It does not cross the placental barrier and thus can be used as an anticoagulant during pregnancy.

196. The answer is D. *(DiPalma, 4/e, pp 422–423. Isselbacher, 13/e, pp 1031–1034. Katzung, 6/e, p 226.)* Although antiarrhythmic drugs are capable of reducing the number of premature ventricular contractions and even eliminating nonsustained ventricular tachycardia, they do not prolong life. This was conclusively shown in the Cardiac Arrhythmia Suppression Trial (CAST), a large-scale study that compared use of antiarrhythmic agents against placebo. Class I antiarrhythmic drugs are apt to cause proarrhythmic changes as well as torsades de pointes. Longevity in cardiac disease is related more closely to the degree of depression of the ejection fraction than to the incidence of arrhythmias.

197. The answer is C. *(DiPalma, 4/e, pp 396–397. Gilman, 8/e, pp 836–837.)* The bipyridines have no relationship to digitalis and do not affect Na^+,K^+-ATPase. They do cause an inhibition of phosphodiesterase III isoenzyme, resulting in an increase in cyclic AMP activity. This causes an increase in protein kinase activity and in calcium influx. Myocardial contractility is enhanced. Unfortunately, bipyridines are suitable only for short-term use.

198. The answer is D. *(DiPalma, 4/e, pp 489–490. Gilman, 8/e, pp 630–631.)* Cromolyn does not relax bronchial or other smooth muscle. In fact it may on rare occasions cause bronchospasm. It is used prophylactically rather than acutely in an asthmatic attack. Cromolyn does reduce bronchial hyperresponsiveness, presumably by inhibiting antigen-induced bronchospasm. The exact role played by its ability to stabilize mast cells is not clear.

199–200. The answers are 199-C, 200-D. *(DiPalma, 4/e, pp 447–449. Gilman, 8/e, pp 881–894.)* Cholestyramine is an anion-exchange resin that is not absorbed. It binds bile acids in the intestine and increases fecal excretion of the acids. Cholestyramine must be combined with a low-cholesterol diet to be effective.

Nicotinic acid is an older drug that decreases the production of VLDL in the liver and lowers the blood level of LDL. The total synthesis of cholesterol in the body is not decreased and nicotinic acid therapy is best combined with other cholesterol-reducing drugs and a low-cholesterol diet. Nicotinic acid does not significantly alter excretion of bile acids. While nicotinic acid does inhibit lipolysis, it also decreases esterification of triglycerides in the liver.

201–202. The answers are 201-A, 202-B. *(DiPalma, 4/e, pp 470–479. Gilman, 8/e, pp 789–808.)* Guanfacine is the newest of a group of drugs including clonidine, guanabenz, and methyldopa that lowers blood pressure by activating brainstem receptors to cause peripheral vasodilation. They are classed as centrally acting sympathetic inhibitors.

The peripherally acting sympathetic inhibitors include all the beta blockers as well as prazosin, terazosin, and doxazosin, which act as alpha$_1$-adrenergic blockers. The latter are very effective in comparison to phentolamine and phenoxybenzamine, which block both alpha$_1$- and alpha$_2$-adrenergic receptors.

203–205. The answers are 203-C, 204-A, 205-E. *(DiPalma, 4/e, pp 118, 122, 398, 490. Gilman, 8/e, pp 161, 173, 798, 813, 1483.)* Isoproterenol, a catecholamine that acts on beta-adrenergic receptors, is given parenterally because absorption after sublingual or oral administration is unreliable. It is a synthetic sympathomimetic structurally similar to epinephrine. Isoproterenol produces myocardial stimulation and is used for the treatment of atrioventricular heart block, cardiogenic shock associated with myocardial infarction, cardiac arrest, and septicemic shock.

Terbutaline is a synthetic sympathomimetic amine that acts on the beta-adrenergic receptors of bronchial smooth muscle and causes a decrease in airway and pulmonary resistance. Oral doses are effective for management of bronchial asthma and for the reversible bronchospasm that may occur in bronchitis and emphysema. Terbutaline has a modest therapeutic advantage over a less selective bronchodilator.

The coronary vasodilator nitroglycerine may be administered orally, sublingually, topically, intravenously, and most recently transdermally. Its small dose and molecular structure permit its passage through the skin. This is accomplished by attaching a nitroglycerine-containing, multilayered film to the skin.

Beclomethasone is a glucocorticoid especially designed for aerosol administration. This permits its therapeutic action in the lungs while minimizing systemic effects. Great care must be exercised when transferring patients from systemic corticosteroids to beclomethasone because fatal adrenal insufficiency has occurred in asthmatic patients undergoing such transfer.

Sodium nitroprusside can only be administered intravenously. It is an effective vasodilator for heart failure because it dilates both arterioles and veins and thus reduces both preload and afterload. Maximal onset of action is in 1 to 2 min, and the effect dissipates rapidly when infusion is stopped.

Cromolyn sodium is inhaled as a powder administered by a special device ("turbo-inhaler").

206–207. The answers are 206-E, 207-A. *(DiPalma, 4/e, pp 430–434. Gilman, 8/e, pp 774–778, 805–806.)* The calcium channel blockers have a diverse chemistry, suggesting different receptor sites. Verapamil is a diphenylalkylamine; diltiazem is a benzothiazepine; bepridil is a pyrrolidine-ethanamine; nifedipine and the others are dihydropyridines. Verapamil is the oldest, and because it has actions on blood vessels and nodal and conduction tissues, it has the most FDA-approved indications.

Amlodipine and nifedipine have actions mostly on blood vessels and therefore have been used mainly for hypertension. In contrast to amlodipine, nifedipine does have some depressant action on cardiac contractility.

208–209. The answers are 208-G, 209-B. *(DiPalma, 4/e, pp 401, 410. Gilman, 8/e, pp 847–849.)* It is widely accepted that antiarrhythmic drugs are best classified according to their electrophysiologic attributes. This is best accomplished by relating the effects of the different drugs to their actions on sodium and calcium channels, which are reflected by changes in the monophasic action potential.

Amiodarone blocks sodium channels and markedly prolongs repolarization, particularly in depolarized cells. Flecainide is related to local anesthetics and also affects sodium channels, but has little effect on repolarization. Mexiletine, which is in the same group of local anesthetics as lidocaine, is remarkable because it either does not affect or shortens repolarization. Its action is mainly on depolarized fibers. Disopyramide slows depolarization and repolarization and, like quinidine, delays conduction. Verapamil, a calcium channel blocker, affects the resting potential or phase 4 and thus has its greatest effect on pacemaker tissue; it is mainly of utility in supraventricular arrhythmias. Digitalis also affects phase 4 of the action potential, but it also greatly hastens repolarization. Although nifedipine is a calcium channel blocker, it has little effect on the electrophysiology of the heart. Propranolol has actions mainly on slow-response fibers and suppresses automaticity.

210–212. The answers are 210-F, 211-E, 212-B. *(DiPalma, 4/e, pp 486–498. Gilman, 8/e, pp 620–635.)* Acetylcholine is the motor for the smooth muscle of the bronchi, and ipratropium appears to inhibit vagally mediated reflexes by antagonizing the action of acetylcholine. Reflex alpha stimuli carried over the vagus nerve cause bronchospasm. Actually ipratropium is of little use in asthma but is effective in chronic obstructive pulmonary disease (COPD).

Acetylcysteine, known as a mucolytic, breaks the fibrillar molecules of mucoproteins by breaking down disulfide bridges of glycoproteins. It is useful in dissolution and expectoration of bronchial inflammatory products.

Cromolyn, a mast cell stabilizer, also inhibits the release of inflammatory agents (leukotrienes) from other inflammatory cells. It has anti-platelet-activating activity as well.

213–215. The answers are 213-C, 214-D, 215-F. *(DiPalma, 4/e, pp 437, 528–530, 533–534, 831–832. Gilman, 8/e, pp 1314–1316,*

1317–1322, 1323–1327.) Coumarin derivatives antagonize vitamin K and cause a decrease in production of prothrombin and coagulation factors VII, IX, and X. Oral anticoagulants prevent formation of these factors by blocking formation of the reduced form of vitamin K.

Dipyridamole is classified as a coronary vasodilator. Its effectiveness in inhibiting platelet aggregation and adhesion has been proved in vitro but has still to be demonstrated in vivo. Dipyridamole is used in patients with prosthetic heart valves as primary prophylaxis against thromboemboli. It is used in combination with warfarin.

Ethylenediaminetetraacetic acid (EDTA) inactivates calcium in vitro by forming a complex with the calcium, thus preventing clotting. This approach is impossible in vivo because calcium levels that are low enough to prevent coagulation also are low enough to be lethal.

216–217. The answers are 216-E, 217-C. *(DiPalma, 4/e, pp 514, 518–519. Gilman, 8/e, pp 1279–1282, 1303–1305.)* Erythropoietin is synthesized mainly by the kidneys. This function is lost in advanced renal disease. Now manufactured by recombinant technology, erythropoietin makes it possible to avoid or greatly reduce the need for blood transfusion in dialysis patients. It is often necessary to also administer iron and folate to prevent deficiency of these factors.

In chronic alcoholism the diet is deficient in folate and other vitamins; the required calories are supplied by alcohol itself. The macrocytic anemia that develops responds best to folic acid therapy.

218–220. The answers are 218-B, 219-D, 220-E. *(DiPalma, 4/e, pp 470, 479–482. Gilman, 8/e, pp 208–209, 749–752.)* The enzyme renin acts upon angiotensinogen (an alpha globulin) to yield the decapeptide angiotensin I, which has limited pharmacologic activity. Angiotensin I is metabolized extensively in a single passage through the lungs by the carboxypeptidase peptidyl dipeptidase (also called *kinase II*, or *angiotensin-converting enzyme*) to the octapeptide angiotensin II.

Angiotensin II has a potent direct action on the vascular smooth muscle and also indirectly stimulates contraction by means of the sympathetic nervous system. The vasoconstriction in response to angiotensin II involves precapillary arterioles and postcapillary venules and results in an increased total peripheral resistance.

The octapeptide saralasin is an analogue of angiotensin II and has an alanine in place of the phenylalanine in the 8 position. It is a potent antagonist of angiotensin II and, thus, can reduce elevated blood pressure in patients with significant amounts of circulating angiotensin II (i.e., renin-dependent hypertension). Being a polypeptide, saralasin must be administered intravenously, which limits its therapeutic use.

Captopril and clonidine, in contrast, are orally effective antihypertensive agents. Captopril (D-3-mercapto-methylpropanoyl-L-proline) is a rationally designed, competitive inhibitor of peptidyl dipeptidase. Unlike saralasin, it blocks the formation but not the response of angiotensin II. Captopril is useful in reducing the blood pressure of both renin-dependent and normal-renin essential hypertension. The hypotensive action of clonidine is believed to be due primarily to stimulation of the alpha-adrenergic receptors in the central nervous system (CNS). A reduction in the discharge rate of preganglionic adrenergic nerves occurs in addition to bradycardia. The CNS actions of clonidine also lead to a reduction in the level of renin activity in the plasma.

221–222. The answers are 221-B, 222-D. *(DiPalma, 4/e, pp 534–536. Gilman, 8/e, pp 732, 738, 1325. Isselbacher, 13/e, pp 1804–1806.)* Desmopressin is a synthetic structural analogue of the pituitary hormone vasopressin. Aside from its antidiuretic function, it stimulates the release from endogenous pools of factor VIII into the circulation, making it useful in mild cases of hemophilia or von Willebrand's disease.

Aminocaproic acid is not an actual procoagulant. It does promote coagulation by acting as a competitive inhibitor of plasminogen binding to fibrin, thus impeding the fibrinolytic mechanism. Oral or parenteral administration is useful in systemic fibrinolysis and urinary fibrinolysis.

Antihemolytic factor, or factor VIII, is missing in hemophiliacs because of an X-linked genetic disorder. Replacing it restores the normal coagulability of blood. Factor IX complex is missing in hemophilia B, and its replacement is required to restore coagulation in these patients. Both factors carry the risk of viral infection.

Oxidized cellulose is a topical agent. On contact with tissue fluids, it becomes an artificial clot and is useful in many types of surgery.

Central Nervous System

- General Anesthetics
  - Halothane*
  - Euflurane*
  - Isoflurane
  - Methoxyflurane
  - Nitrous oxide
  - Desflurane
  - Sevoflurane
- Intravenous Anesthetics
  - Thiopental*
  - Methohexital
  - Midazolam
  - Ketamine
  - Etomidate
  - Fentanyl
  - Propofol
- Sedatives and Hypnotics
  - Barbiturates
    - Amobarbital
    - Butabarbital
    - Secobarbital
    - Mephobarbital
    - Metharbital
    - Phenobarbital*
  - Benzodiazepines
    - Flurazepam*
    - Temazepam
    - Triazolam
    - Quazepam
    - Estazolam
  - Miscellaneous group
    - Chloral hydrate
    - Paraldehyde
    - Ethchlorvynol
    - Ethinamate
    - Glutethimide
    - Zolpidem
- Antianxiety Drugs
  - Benzodiazepines
    - Chlordiazepoxide*
    - Diazepam*
    - Clorazepate
    - Halazepam
    - Lorazepam
    - Oxazepam
    - Prazepam
    - Alprazolam
  - Propanediols
    - Meprobamate*
  - Miscellaneous
    - Buspirone
    - Hydroxyzine
- Ethanol and Related Alcohols
  - Ethanol*
  - Ethylene glycol
  - Isopropyl alcohol
  - Methanol
  - Disulfiram as a deterrent
- Psychotomimetic Drugs
  - Lysergic acid diethylamide (LSD)*
  - Mescaline
  - Psilocybin
  - Phencyclidine
  - Amphetamine
  - Methamphetamine
  - Cocaine*

- Marijuana*
- Antipsychotic Drugs
  - Phenothiazines
    - Promazine
    - Chlorpromazine*
    - Triflupromazine
    - Prochlorperazine
    - Trifluoperazine
    - Fluphenazine
    - Thioridazine
  - Thioxanthene derivatives
    - Chlorprothixene
    - Thiothixene
  - Butyrophenone
    - Haloperidol*
  - Miscellaneous group
    - Molindone
    - Loxapine
    - Pimozide
    - Lithium carbonate
- Antidepressant Drugs
  - Tricyclics
    - Imipramine*
    - Amitriptyline
    - Desipramine
    - Nortriptyline
    - Protriptyline
    - Trimipramine
    - Doxepin
  - Monoamine oxidase inhibitors
    - Tranylcypromine*
    - Phenelzine
    - Isocarboxazid
  - Second-generation antidepressants
    - Maprotiline
    - Amoxapine
    - Trazodone
    - Fluoxetine*
    - Sertraline
    - Paroxetine
- Antiepileptic and Antiparkinsonism Drugs
  - Tonic-clonic and focal seizures
    - Phenytoin,* mephenytoin
    - Carbamazepine
    - Phenobarbital
    - Primidone
  - Absence seizures
    - Ethosuximide*
    - Valproic acid*
    - Clonazepam
    - Trimethadione
    - Gabapentin
  - Anticholinergics for parkinsonism
    - Trihexyphenidyl*
    - Procyclidine
    - Biperiden
    - Benztropine*
    - Diphenhydramine
    - Orpehadrine
  - Levodopa for parkinsonism
    - Selegiline*
  - Miscellaneous agents for parkinsonism
    - Amantadine
    - Bromocriptine*
- Narcotic Analgesics
  - Endogenous opioid peptides
    - Met- and leu-enkephalin
    - β-Endorphin
    - Dynorphin
  - Agonists
    - Morphine*
    - Codeine*
    - Heroin
    - Hydromorphone
    - Oxymorphone
    - Oxycodone
    - Levorphanol
    - Meperidine, methadone
    - Propoxyphene
  - Antagonists
    - Naloxone*
    - Naltrexone*

- Mixed agonists-antagonists
  - Buprenorphine
  - Butorphanol
  - Nalbuphine
  - Pentazocine
  - Dezocine
- Local Anesthetics
  - Esters
    - Cocaine*
    - Procaine*
    - Chloroprocaine
    - Tetracaine
  - Amides
    - Lidocaine*
    - Mepivacaine
    - Bupivacine
    - Etidocaine
    - Prilocaine
- Drug Dependence
  - Terms
    - Psychological dependence
    - Addiction
    - Physical dependence
    - Drug abuse
    - Tolerance
  - Schedules of Drug Enforcement Administration
    - Numbers I to VI
  - Stimulants
    - Cocaine and amphetamines
    - Hallucinogens (LSD)
    - Marijuana

DIRECTIONS: Each question below contains five suggested responses. Select the **one best** response to each question.

223. Which of the following antidepressants has its mechanism of action primarily associated with blockade of serotonin uptake?

(A) Imipramine
(B) Nortriptyline
(C) Fluoxetine
(D) Desipramine
(E) Doxepin

224. Which of the following opioid agonists is only administered by the parenteral route?

(A) Morphine
(B) Codeine
(C) Fentanyl
(D) Methadone
(E) Propoxyphene

225. Which of the following local anesthetics is useful for topical (surface) administration only?

(A) Procaine
(B) Bupivacaine
(C) Etidocaine
(D) Benzocaine
(E) Lidocaine

226. Akathisia, Parkinson-like syndrome, galactorrhea, and amenorrhea are side effects of perphenazine caused by

(A) blockade of muscarinic receptors
(B) blockade of alpha-adrenergic receptors
(C) blockade of dopamine receptors
(D) supersensitivity of dopamine receptors
(E) stimulation of nicotinic receptors

227. Which of the following agents is useful in treatment of malignant hyperthermia?

(A) Baclofen
(B) Diazepam
(C) Cyclobenzaprine
(D) Dantrolene
(E) Halothane

228. Inhibitors of serotonin uptake like paroxetine interact significantly with which of the following drugs?

(A) Chlorpromazine
(B) Tranylcypromine
(C) Halothane
(D) Benztropine
(E) Digitalis

229. Which of the following is an antidepressant agent that selectively inhibits serotonin (5-HT) uptake with minimal effect on norepinephrine uptake?

(A) Protriptyline
(B) Maprotiline
(C) Fluoxetine
(D) Desipramine
(E) Amoxapine

230. Which of the following inhalation anesthetics is most likely to produce hepatotoxicity?

(A) Isoflurane
(B) Enflurane
(C) Methoxyfluane
(D) Halothane
(E) Nitrous oxide

231. Carbidopa is useful in the treatment of Parkinson's disease because it

(A) is a precursor of L-dopa
(B) is a dopaminergic receptor agonist
(C) prevents peripheral biotransformation of L-dopa
(D) prevents breakdown of dopamine
(E) promotes a decreased concentration of L-dopa in the nigrostriatum

232. Which of the following is described as a competitive benzodiazepine receptor antagonist?

(A) Ketamine
(B) Chlordiazepoxide
(C) Flumazenil
(D) Midazolam
(E) Triazolam

233. Which of the following drugs mimics the activity of metenkephalin in the dorsal horn of the spinal cord?

(A) Selegiline
(B) Trihexyphenidyl
(C) Baclofen
(D) Morphine
(E) Phenobarbital

234. The preferred treatment of status epilepticus is intravenous administration of

(A) chlorpromazine
(B) diazepam
(C) succinylcholine
(D) tranylcypromine
(E) ethosuximide

235. The most common adverse effect associated with the tricyclic antidepressants is

(A) anticholinergic effects
(B) seizures
(C) arrhythmias
(D) hepatotoxicity
(E) nephrotoxicity

236. Which of the following statements correctly characterizes benzodiazepines?

(A) They are considered nonspecific central nervous system depressants
(B) They increase the frequency of chloride ion channel openings
(C) They increase the time of chloride ion channel opening
(D) They increase the activity of dopamine on chloride channels
(E) They increase the activity of sodium channels

237. Which of the following is a selective inhibitor of monoamine oxidase B useful in the treatment of parkinsonism?

(A) Bromocriptine
(B) Carbidopa
(C) Deprenyl (selegiline)
(D) Phenelzine
(E) Tranylcypromine

238. Which of the following statements is true concerning abuse of opioid analgesics?

(A) No cross tolerance develops among opioid analgesics
(B) Tolerance develops equally to all effects of opioids
(C) Opioids reduce pain, aggression, and sexual drives
(D) The symptoms of acute methadone withdrawal are qualitatively different from those of acute heroin withdrawal
(E) None of the above

239. Neuroleptic malignant syndrome is associated with use of

(A) oxazepam (Serax)
(B) amobarbital (Amytal)
(C) doxepin hydrochloride (Sinequan)
(D) trifluoperazine hydrochloride (Stelazine)
(E) phenytoin (Dilantin)

240. A drug that specifically enhances metabolically the activity of brain dopamine is

(A) benztropine
(B) selegiline
(C) trihexyphenidyl
(D) bromocriptine
(E) chlorpromazine

241. A dopamine receptor agonist useful in the therapy of Parkinson's disease is

(A) selegiline
(B) bromocriptine
(C) apomorphine
(D) amantidine
(E) belladonna

242. In addition to its use in the treatment of schizophrenia, chlorpromazine (Thorazine) is effective

(A) in reducing nausea and vomiting
(B) as in antihypertensive agent
(C) as an anthistaminic
(D) in the treatment of depression
(E) for treating bipolar affective disorder

243. Morphine may be best characterized by which of the following statements?

(A) It is classified as a mixed agonist-antagonist drug
(B) It inhibits withdrawal symptoms in persons dependent on heroin
(C) At high doses it causes death by respiratory depression
(D) It is a pure opioid antagonist at the mu, kappa, and delta receptors
(E) It has an addiction potential equal to that of codeine

244. Cocaine, produced from the leaves of *Erythroxylon* species,

(A) produces bradycardia and vasodilation
(B) is directly related chemically to opioid analgesics
(C) is metabolized by the microsomal metabolizing system
(D) effectively blocks nerve conduction
(E) blocks norepinephrine receptors directly

245. A drug of choice for the therapy of absence seizures is

(A) phenobarbital
(B) phenytoin
(C) carbamazepine
(D) ethosuximide
(E) trimethadione

246. Which of the following agents is a selective D_2 (dopamine receptor) agonist?

(A) Fluphenazine
(B) Bromocriptine
(C) Promethazine
(D) Haloperidol
(E) Chlorpromazine

247. Haloperidol may best be characterized by which of the following statements?

(A) It is classified as a phenothiazine
(B) It is a selective D_2 receptor agonist
(C) Its mechanism of action is completely different from that of chlorpromazine
(D) It is more potent as an antipsychotic drug than is chlorpromazine
(E) It produces a lower incidence of extrapyramidal reactions than does chlorpromazine

248. A correct statement regarding alprazolam is that it

(A) potentiates the activity of dopamine as its major mechanism of action
(B) is more potent than diazepam in relieving skeletal muscle spasm
(C) is useful in the management of anxiety
(D) causes more severe respiratory depression than does phenobarbital
(E) is classified as a long-acting phenothiazine derivative

249. Phencyclidine may best be characterized by which of the following statements?

(A) It has opioid activity
(B) Its mechanism of action is related to its anticholinergic properties
(C) It can cause significant hallucinogenic activity
(D) It causes significant withdrawal symptoms
(E) Treatment of overdose is with an opiate

250. Which of the following statements about "crack" (the free-base form of cocaine) is true?

(A) "Flashbacks" (recurrences of effects) may occur months after the last use of the drug
(B) It may cause seizures and cardiac arrhythmias
(C) It acts by blocking adrenergic receptors
(D) It is the salt form of cocaine
(E) It is primarily administered intranasally

DIRECTIONS: Each numbered question or incomplete statement below is NEGATIVELY phrased. Select the **one best** lettered response.

251. All the following compounds are indicated for the treatment of psychoses EXCEPT

(A) perphenazine (Trilafon)
(B) thiothixene hydrochloride (Navane)
(C) fluoxetine hydrochloride (Prozac)
(D) haloperidol (Haldol)
(E) loxapine succinate (Loxitane)

252. Triazolam, a central nervous system depressant, is characterized by all the following statements EXCEPT

(A) it binds to benzodiazepine receptor, enhancing GABA-mediated chloride influx
(B) it is useful in the treatment of insomnia
(C) it enhances the activity of the drug-metabolizing microsomal system
(D) combined with ethanol, it may produce significant respiratory depression
(E) adverse effects may include drowsiness, dizziness, lethargy, and ataxia

253. All the statements that follow accurately describe the pharmacology of lidocaine EXCEPT

(A) it acts by interfering with sodium influx in nerve fibers
(B) coadministration of epinephrine would prolong its duration of action
(C) adverse reactions to its use may include CNS and cardiovascular depression
(D) it is biotransformed by plasma esterases
(E) it is slowly metabolized in the fetus and neonate

254. All the following benzodiazepines are biotransformed to active products EXCEPT

(A) alprazolam
(B) diazepam
(C) oxazepam
(D) prazepam
(E) chlordiazepoxide

255. Effects of thioridazine include all the following EXCEPT

(A) orthostatic hypotension, constipation, and urinary retention
(B) tardive dyskinesia
(C) hypoprolactinemia
(D) antiemesis
(E) control of psychotic behavior

256. Flurazepam has all the following characteristics EXCEPT

(A) classification as a benzodiazepine
(B) primary use as a hypnotic
(C) production of physical dependence
(D) effective production of analgesia
(E) long duration of action (greater than 24 h)

257. A high degree of tolerance develops to all the following effects of hydromorphone EXCEPT

(A) euphoria
(B) analgesia
(C) nausea and vomiting
(D) respiratory depression
(E) constipation

258. All the following statements about methadone are true EXCEPT

(A) it is useful as an analgesic
(B) it has greater oral efficacy than morphine
(C) it possesses opioid antagonist effects
(D) it produces a milder but more protracted withdrawal syndrome than that associated with morphine
(E) adverse reactions may include constipation, respiratory depression, and lightheadedness

259. All the following statements are true about amphetamine EXCEPT that it

(A) releases catecholamines from central and peripheral adrenergic neurons
(B) may cause tachycardia, cardiac arrhythmias, and anginal pain
(C) is used in the treatment of narcolepsy
(D) is rapidly biotransformed by catechol-*O*-methyltransferase (COMT)
(E) can lead to toxic psychosis, hyperthermia, and hypertension

260. Desipramine can produce all the following EXCEPT

(A) sedation
(B) xerostomia and constipation
(C) anticonvulsant effect
(D) orthostatic hypotension
(E) decrease in REM sleep

261. Thiopental is used as a general anesthetic. All the following statements characterize its actions EXCEPT

(A) it is ultra-short-acting by virtue of redistribution
(B) it sensitizes the myocardium to endogenous catecholamines
(C) it may cause laryngospasm and bronchospasm
(D) it is biotransformed to pentobarbital
(E) it produces little postanesthetic excitement or vomiting

262. All the following are typical toxicities of ethanol EXCEPT

(A) it is a hepatotoxic agent
(B) it elevates body temperature by peripheral vasoconstriction
(C) it suppresses the release of antidiuretic hormone
(D) it can lead to gastritis and pancreatitis
(E) acute overdose can cause acidosis, hypoglycemia, and elevated intracranial pressure

263. All the following statements regarding the effects of amitriptyline are true EXCEPT

(A) it causes significant sedation
(B) it possesses anticholinergic effects
(C) its mechanism of action is primarily associated with blockade of serotonin but not norepinephrine uptake
(D) it stimulates GABA receptors
(E) it has a high potential for causing orthostatic hypotension

264. Lidocaine (Xylocaine), a commonly used local anesthetic, has all the following effects EXCEPT

(A) it is biotransformed by amidase
(B) vasodilation increases duration of action
(C) it has rapid onset of action
(D) topical application can produce surface anesthesia
(E) it can be used to induce epidural anesthesia

265. Clorazepate has all the following attributes EXCEPT

(A) it may cause psychological dependence
(B) it is activated in the stomach
(C) it is useful as an antianxiety agent
(D) it has a duration of action of less than 10 h
(E) its onset of action is rapid

266. Benzodiazepine derivatives have a wide variety of central nervous system activity, including all the following EXCEPT

(A) flurazepam is useful for insomnia
(B) diazepam is useful for symptoms of acute alcohol withdrawal
(C) lorazepam is useful as a premedication for endoscopy
(D) clonazepam is useful for generalized tonic-clonic seizures
(E) chlordiazepoxide is useful as a long-acting antianxiety agent

267. Phenytoin's activities include all the following EXCEPT

(A) it appears to suppress the spread of neuronal discharge from an initiating site adjacent to remote brain areas
(B) plasma protein binding is greater than 90 percent
(C) its major use is in the treatment of absence seizures
(D) its major side effect is ataxia
(E) it can cause hyperplasia of the gums

268. All the following are characteristics of lithium carbonate EXCEPT that it

(A) has a general sedation action similar to that of the phenothiazine derivatives
(B) may induce tremors and nephrogenic diabetes insipidus
(C) is useful in the treatment of bipolar affective (manic-depressive) disorders
(D) has a low therapeutic index, and plasma or serum concentrations must be determined to facilitate safe use of the drug
(E) will accumulate in patients who are taking any diuretic that will cause significant Na^+ depletion

269. All the following agents enhance the activity of γ-aminobutyric acid (GABA) EXCEPT

(A) chlordiazepoxide
(B) phenobarbital
(C) halazepam
(D) valproic acid
(E) chlorpromazine

270. Marijuana, an addicting drug, has all the following characteristics EXCEPT

(A) it may lower intraocular pressure
(B) a sign of acute intoxication is reddening of conjunctiva
(C) it has antiemetic properties
(D) heavy chronic use can lower serum testosterone levels in men
(E) it causes flashbacks

271. All the following drugs produce an abstinence syndrome characterized as being excitatory EXCEPT

(A) morphine
(B) ethanol
(C) phenobarbital
(D) cocaine
(E) glutethimide

272. Naltrexone, a widely used agent in the rehabilitation of opioid-dependent patients, has all the following characteristics EXCEPT

(A) it lacks opioid agonist activity at therapeutic doses
(B) it possesses longer duration of action than naloxone
(C) it will precipitate withdrawal syndrome in a heroin addict
(D) it is usually administered intravenously
(E) it is subject to "first-pass" metabolism in the liver

273. Drugs that produce their pharmacologic effects by inhibition of prostaglandin synthesis include all the following EXCEPT

(A) indomethacin
(B) ibuprofen
(C) acetaminophen
(D) piroxicam
(E) naproxen

274. All the following are a consequence of ethanol abuse EXCEPT

(A) development of metabolic tolerance
(B) reduced effect of barbiturates in an intoxicated alcoholic person
(C) possible development of disorientation, tremors, hallucinations, and convulsions when consumption of ethanol is abruptly ended
(D) hepatitis
(E) pancreatitis

275. Barbiturates, in addition to their sedative effects, have all the following characteristics EXCEPT

(A) pentobarbital is a biotransformation product of thiopental
(B) phenobarbital can decrease the enzymatic activity of δ-aminolevulinic acid
(C) mephobarbital can be used in the treatment of tonic-clonic seizures
(D) the duration of effect for methohexital is determined by redistribution
(E) alkalinization of the urine readily enhances the excretion of secobarbital

276. Correct statements concerning fentanyl include all the following EXCEPT

(A) it has been shown to be up to 100 times more potent than morphine
(B) it is usually administered orally
(C) it is useful for anesthesia
(D) at high doses it produces muscular rigidity, which is reversed by naloxone
(E) it is combined with droperidol to produce neuroleptanalgesia

277. The general anesthetic halothane (Fluothane) has all the following characteristics EXCEPT

(A) it is more potent as an anesthetic than nitrous oxide
(B) it increases cardiac output
(C) it causes respiratory depression with increased anesthetic levels
(D) it may produce hepatotoxicity
(E) it is a halogenated alkane

278. The mechanisms of drugs used in the therapy of parkinsonism include all the following EXCEPT

(A) benztropine blocks muscarinic receptors
(B) amantadine stimulates release of dopamine from storage sites
(C) bromocriptine stimulates dopaminergic receptors
(D) levodopa enhances the synthesis of dopamine
(E) selegiline is an inhibitor of monoamine oxidase A

279. Codeine, a commonly used opiate, is accurately described by all the following statements EXCEPT

(A) it produces naloxone-reversible respiratory depression
(B) it may cause hypotension as a result of histamine release
(C) it has antitussive properties
(D) it is exempt from the narcotics control laws
(E) it is partially biotransformed to morphine

280. Naloxone, an opiate antagonist, has all the following characteristics EXCEPT

(A) it reverses the analgesic effects of butorphanol
(B) it is useful for the treatment of opiate overdose
(C) it induces withdrawal symptoms in a heroin addict
(D) it reverses phenobarbital-induced respiratory depression
(E) it has poor oral bioavailability

DIRECTIONS: Each group of questions below consists of lettered headings followed by a set of numbered items. For each numbered item select the **one** lettered heading with which it is **most** closely associated. Each lettered heading may be used **once, more than once, or not at all.**

Questions 281–283

Match each description with the appropriate drug.

(A) Isocarboxazid (Marplan)
(B) Trazodone (Desyrel)
(C) Mesoridazine (Serentil)
(D) Pimozide (Orap)
(E) Amitriptyline (Elavil)
(F) Fluoxetine (Prozac)
(G) Protriptyline (Vivactil)
(H) Amoxapine (Asendin)
(I) Clozapine (Clozaril)
(J) Nortriptyline (Aventyl)
(K) Fluphenazine (Prolixin)
(L) Molindone (Moban)

281. This tricyclic antidepressant has high anticholinergic activity, is one of the more sedating compounds of the group, and is biotransformed to a long-acting active product.

282. Relatively insoluble salts of this antipsychotic drug have been prepared for use as intramuscular depot injections

283. This drug has the lowest incidence of extrapyramidal reactions, but the highest incidence of agranulocytosis, of all the antipsychotic compounds

Questions 284–286

Match each description with the appropriate drug.

(A) Primidone
(B) Disulfiram
(C) Dextroamphetamine
(D) Valproic acid
(E) Flurazepam
(F) Phenylephrine
(G) Phenytoin
(H) Isoetharine
(I) Carbamazepine
(J) Amitriptyline
(K) Triazolam
(L) Diazepam

284. Causes megaloblastic anemia, ataxia, and gingival hyperplasia

285. Is used in the management of ethanol withdrawal, as a preanesthetic medication, and in the treatment of status epilepticus

286. May cause increased alertness, elevated mood states, insomnia, irritability, and hallucinations

Questions 287–289

Many drugs are associated with an ability to induce physical dependence as well as a craving for and tolerance to their psychological effects. For each of the drugs listed below, choose the effect that it usually produces.

(A) Psychic dependence
(B) Tachyphylaxis
(C) Physical dependence only
(D) Tolerance and physical dependence
(E) Hallucinations
(F) Psychedelic effects
(G) Low potential of addiction

287. Meperidine

288. Secobarbital

289. Chlorpromazine

Central Nervous System

Answers

223. The answer is C. *(DiPalma, 4/e, pp 289–291. Gilman, 8/e, pp 407–410.)* Tricyclic antidepressants block the reuptake of norepinephrine and serotonin into the presynaptic nerve terminal. Fluoxetine, sertraline, and paroxetine work primarily by inhibiting serotonin uptake and have little or no effect on blockade of norepinephrine into the presynaptic nerve terminal.

224. The answer is C. *(DiPalma, 4/e, p 327. Gilman, 8/e, pp 303–306.)* Fentanyl is a chemical relative of meperidine that is nearly 100 times more potent than morphine. The duration of action, usually between 30 and 60 min after parenteral administration, is shorter than that of meperidine. Fentanyl citrate is only available for parenteral administration intramuscularly and intravenously.

225. The answer is D. *(DiPalma, 4/e, pp 365–371, 373. Gilman, 8/e, p 321.)* Local anesthetics are agents that, when applied locally, block nerve conduction; they also prevent generation of a nerve impulse. All contain a lipophilic (benzene) functional group and most a hydrophilic (amine) group. Benzocaine does not contain the terminal hydrophilic amine group; thus, it is only slightly soluble in water and is slowly absorbed with a prolonged duration. It is, therefore, only useful as a surface anesthetic.

226. The answer is C. *(DiPalma, 4/e, pp 275–282. Gilman, 8/e, pp 383–399.)* Unwanted pharmacologic side effects produced by phenothiazine antipsychotic drugs (e.g., perphenazine) include Parkinson-like syndrome, akathisia, dystonias, galactorrhea, amenorrhea, and infertility. These side effects are due to the ability of these agents to block dopamine receptors. The phenothiazines also block muscarinic and alpha-adrenergic receptors, which are responsible for other effects.

227. The answer is D. *(DiPalma, 4/e, pp 225–226. Gilman, 8/e, pp 480–481.)* Malignant hyperthermia (hyperpyrexia), a syndrome associated with use of a general anesthetic (e.g., halothane) in conjunction with a skeletal muscle relaxant, is characterized by tachycardia, hyperventilation, arrhythmias, fever, muscular fasciculation, and rigidity. It is caused by a sudden increase in the availability of calcium ions in the myoplasma of muscle. Dantrolene, which interferes with release of calcium ions from the sarcoplasmic reticulum, is indicated in treatment of the disorder. The first three agents are centrally acting skeletal muscle relaxants that are not useful in the treatment of malignant hyperthermia.

228. The answer is B. *(DiPalma, 4/e, p 298. Katzung, 6/e, p 992.)* Fatalities have been reported when fluoxetine and monoamine oxidase inhibitors such as tranylcypromine have been given simultaneously. Monoamine oxidase inhibitors should be stopped at least 2 weeks prior to the administration of fluoxetine or paroxetine. The mechanism of this interaction is under investigation.

229. The answer is C. *(DiPalma, 4/e, p 290. Gilman, 8/e, pp 405–406.)* The tricyclics and second-generation antidepressants act by blocking serotonin or norepinephrine uptake into the presynaptic terminal. Fluoxetine selectively inhibits serotonin uptake with minimal effects on norepinephrine uptake. Protriptyline, maprotiline, desipramine, and amoxapine have greater effect on norepinephrine uptake.

230. The answer is D. *(DiPalma, 4/e, pp 224–225. Gilman, 8/e, pp 286–292.)* Halothane is a substituted alkane general anesthetic. It undergoes significant metabolism in humans with about 20 percent of the absorbed dose recovered as metabolites. Halothane can cause postoperative jaundice and hepatic necrosis with repeated administration in rare instances.

231. The answer is C. *(DiPalma, 4/e, pp 314–316. Gilman, 8/e, p 471.)* Carbidopa is an inhibitor of aromatic L-amino acid decarboxylase. It cannot readily penetrate the CNS and thus decreases the decarboxylation of L-dopa in the peripheral tissues. This promotes an increased concentration of L-dopa in the nigrostriatum, where it is converted to dopamine. In addition, the effective dose of levodopa can be reduced.

232. The answer is C. *(DiPalma, 4/e, p 232. Katzung, 6/e, p 342.)* Flumazenil is a competitive benzodiazepine receptor antagonist. The drug reverses the CNS sedative effects of benzodiazepines and is indicated where general anesthesia has been induced by or maintained with benzodiazepines such as diazepam, lorazepam, or midazolam.

233. The answer is D. *(DiPalma, 4/e, pp 319–324. Gilman, 8/e, pp 486–487.)* The enkephalins are endogenous agonists of the opioid receptors. They are located in areas of the brain and spinal cord related to the perception of pain. These areas include the laminae I and II of the spinal cord, the spinal trigeminal nucleus, and the periaqueductal gray. Selegiline and trihexyphenidyl are anti-parkinsonism drugs; baclofen is a skeletal muscle relaxant agonist for the γ-aminobutyric acid (GABA) receptor.

234. The answer is B. *(DiPalma, 4/e, pp 250–251. Gilman, 8/e, p 459.)* Intravenously administered diazepam is the drug of choice for treatment of status epilepticus. Diazepam increases the apparent affinity of the inhibitory neurotransmitter γ-aminobutyric acid (GABA) for binding sites on brain cell membranes. The effects of diazepam are short-lasting. Continuing therapy is usually with phenytoin. Other drugs suggested for use in status epilepticus are lorazepam and lidocaine. None of the other drugs listed in the question are appropriate for status epilepticus: chlorpromazine is an antipsychotic; succinylcholine is a neuromuscular blocking agent; tranylcypromine is an antidepressant; ethosuximide is used in petit mal epilepsy.

235. The answer is A. *(DiPalma, 4/e, pp 294–296. Gilman, 8/e, pp 405–414.)* The most common side effects associated with antidepressants are their antimuscarinic effects, which may be evident in over 50 percent of patients. Clinically, the antimuscarinic effects may manifest as dry mouth, blurred vision, constipation, tachycardia, dizziness, and urinary retention. At therapeutic plasma concentrations these drugs usually do not cause changes in the ECG. Direct cardiac effects of the tricyclic antidepressants are important in overdosage.

236. The answer is B. *(DiPalma, 4/e, pp 244–246. Gilman, 8/e, pp 424–427.)* Benzodiazepines are believed to exert their effects through an interaction with a specific site on chloride channels. Stimulation by GABA of $GABA_A$ receptors on the protein complex leads to an increased influx of chloride ions. Benzodiazepines are thought to bind to one site and cause an allosteric change in the protein complex, resulting in an increased frequency of chloride ion channel openings.

237. The answer is C. *(DiPalma, 4/e, pp 315–318. Katzung, 6/e, pp 450–451.)* Two types of monoamine oxidase (MAO) have been found: MAO-A, which metabolizes norepinephrine and serotonin, and MAO-B, which metabolizes dopamine. Deprenyl (selegiline) is a selective inhibitor of MAO-B. It therefore inhibits the breakdown of dopamine and prolongs the therapeutic effectiveness of levodopa in parkinsonism. Bromocriptine is a dopamine receptor agonist. Carbidopa inhibits the peripheral metabolism of levodopa. Both are useful in treatment of parkinsonism. Phenelzine and tranylcypromine are nonselective MAO inhibitors. Combining them with levodopa may lead to hypertensive crises, and thus they are not used in the therapy of parkinsonism.

238. The answer is C. *(DiPalma, 4/e, pp 375–378. Gilman, 8/e, pp 495–504.)* In opioid abuse, there is always a high degree of cross tolerance to other drugs with a similar pharmacologic action even if the chemical composition of the opioids is totally different. Tolerance develops at different rates to different effects of opioids. With methadone, abrupt withdrawal causes a syndrome that is qualitatively similar to that of morphine but is longer and less intense, thus following the general rule that a drug with a shorter duration of action produces a shorter, more intense withdrawal syndrome. The crimes associated with narcotic abuse are considered to be motivated by the need to acquire the drug and not from the effects of the drug per se. Significant tolerance develops to most of the effects of narcotics except for constipation and pinpoint pupils, to which there is minimal tolerance.

239. The answer is D. *(DiPalma, 4/e, pp 280–281. Gilman, 8/e, p 399.)* Neuroleptic malignant syndrome is a condition characterized by hyperthermia, skeletal muscle hypertonicity, catatonia, elevated serum creatinine phosphokinase, fluctuations in consciousness, and labile heart rate and blood pressure. It is a relatively rare adverse reaction to potent antipsychotic drugs, such as trifluoperazine hydrochloride, especially when administered parenterally. Although the prevalence is estimated to be approximately 0.5 to 1 percent of those treated with antipsychotics, the mortality may be as high as 20 percent. This condition is treated by discontinuation of the antipsychotic drug and administration of dantrolene (Dantrium) intravenously (until the symptoms subside and the patient can swallow), then orally; bromocriptine (Parlodel) is added to the therapy. This disorder has not been associated with antianxiety agents (e.g., oxazepam), sedative-hypnotics (e.g., amobarbital), antidepressants (e.g., doxepin hydrochloride), or antiepileptics (e.g., phenytoin).

240. The answer is B. *(DiPalma, 4/e, p 318. Gilman, 8/e, p 475.)* Selegiline inhibits monoamine oxidase B, thus delaying the metabolic breakdown of dopamine. It is effective alone in parkinsonism and increases the effectiveness of levodopa. Benztropine and trihexyphenidyl are cholinergic antagonists in the brain; bromocriptine is a dopamine receptor agonist. Chlorpromazine is an antipsychotic drug with antiadrenergic properties.

241. The answer is B. *(DiPalma, 4/e, pp 317–318. Katzung, 6/e, pp 424–425.)* Bromocriptine mimics the action of dopamine in the brain but is not as readily metabolized. It is especially useful in parkinsonism that is unresponsive to levodopa. Apomorphine is also a dopamine receptor agonist, but its side effects preclude its use for this purpose. Selegiline is a monoamine oxidase inhibitor (type B); atropine is a belladonna preparation; and amantidine is an antiviral agent that probably affects the synthesis or uptake of dopamine.

242. The answer is A. *(DiPalma, 4/e, pp 275–277. Isselbacher, 13/e, pp 2417–2418.)* Chlorpromazine is the prototype compound of the phenothiazine class of antipsychotic drugs. It is indicated for use in the treatment of a variety of psychoses, which includes schizophrenia, and in the treatment of nausea and vomiting, in both adults and children, from a number of causes. The drug can be administered orally, rectally, or intramuscularly for this purpose. It is believed that the effectiveness of the compound is based on inhibition of dopaminergic receptors in the chemoreceptor trigger zone of the medulla. Other phenothiazine derivatives are also used for emesis, including thiethylperazine (Torecan), prochlorperazine (Compazine), and perphenazine (Trilafon). Although chlorpromazine may cause orthostatic hypotension and has mild H_1-histamine receptor blocking activity, the drug is never used as an antihypertensive or as an antihistaminic. Chlorpromazine is not an effective antidepressant drug and lithium salts are used for treating the mania associated with bipolar affective disorder.

243. The answer is C. *(DiPalma, 4/e, pp 325–333. Gilman, 8/e, pp 489–496.)* Morphine is a pure agonist opioid drug with agonist activity toward all the opioid subtype receptor sites. In high doses, deaths associated with morphine are related to the depression of the respiratory center in the medulla. Morphine has a high addiction potential related to the activity of heroin or dihydromorphine. Codeine has a significantly lower addiction potential.

244. The answer is D. *(DiPalma, 4/e, pp 269–270. Gilman, 8/e, pp 319–320.)* Cocaine has local anesthetic properties; it can block the initiation or conduction of a nerve impulse. It is biotransformed by plasma esterases to inactive products. In addition, cocaine blocks the reuptake of norepinephrine. This action produces CNS stimulant effects including euphoria, excitement, and restlessness. Peripherally, cocaine produces sympathomimetic effects including tachycardia and vasoconstriction. Death from acute overdose can be from respiratory depression or cardiac failure. Cocaine is an ester of benzoic acid and closely related to the structure of atropine.

245. The answer is D. *(DiPalma, 4/e, pp 305–313. Gilman, 8/e, pp 449–453.)* Both ethosuximide and valproic acid are used to treat absence seizures. Ethosuximide is more effective than valproic acid for this purpose and exhibits fewer serious adverse effects. Valproic acid has been reported to cause hepatotoxicity. Carbamazepine is effective in the treatment of trigeminal neuralgia and all types of epilepsy except absence seizures. Phenobarbital and phenytoin are effective agents for generalized tonic-clonic and cortical focal seizures. Trimethadione, originally the special drug for absence seizures, is no longer the first choice because of its severe toxicity.

246. The answer is B. *(DiPalma, 4/e, pp 275–277, 317. Gilman, 8/e, p 942.)* Central dopamine receptors are divided into D_1 and D_2 receptors. Antipsychotic activity is better correlated to blockade of D_2 receptors. Haloperidol, a potent antipsychotic, selectively antagonizes at D_2 receptors. Phenothiazine derivatives, such as chlorpromazine, fluphenazine, and promethazine, are not selective for D_2 receptors. Bromocriptine, a selective D_2 agonist, is useful in the treatment of parkinsonism and hyperprolactinemia. It produces fewer adverse reactions than do nonselective dopamine receptor agonists.

247. The answer is D. *(DiPalma, 4/e, p 283. Gilman, 8/e, pp 401–404.)* Haloperidol is a butyrophenone derivative with the same mechanism of action as the phenothiazines, that is, blockade of dopaminergic receptors. It is more selective for D_2 receptors. Haloperidol is more potent on a weight basis than the phenothiazines, but produces a higher incidence of extrapyramidal reactions than does chlorpromazine.

248. The answer is C. *(DiPalma, 4/e, pp 244–251. Katzung, 6/e, pp 343–345.)* Alprazolam is a benzodiazepine derivative classified as an antianxiety agent. It acts by potentiating the activity of GABA. On a weight basis, it is the most potent antianxiety agent. Of the benzodiazepines, only diazepam is useful in relief of skeletal muscle spasm. The benzodiazepines, administered orally, produce only mild respiratory depression; barbiturates have significant depressant effects. Combining benzodiazepines with other CNS depressants (e.g., ethanol) can cause significant respiratory depression.

249. The answer is C. *(DiPalma, 4/e, pp 381–382. Gilman, 8/e, pp 557–558.)* Phencyclidine is a hallucinogenic compound with no opioid activity. Its mechanism of action is amphetamine-like. A withdrawal syndrome has not been described for this drug in human subjects. In overdose the treatment of choice for the psychotic activity is the antipsychotic drug haloperidol.

250. The answer is B. *(DiPalma, 4/e, pp 380–381. Katzung, 6/e, p 483.)* "Crack" is the free-base form (nonsalt form) of the alkaloid cocaine. It is called crack because when heated it makes a crackling sound. Heating crack enables a person to smoke it; the drug is readily absorbed through the lungs and produces an intense euphoric effect in seconds. Use has led to seizures and cardiac arrhythmias. Some of cocaine's effects (sympathomimetic) are due to blockade of norepinephrine reuptake into presynaptic terminals; it does not block receptors. "Flashbacks" can occur with use of LSD and mescaline but have not been associated with the use of cocaine.

251. The answer is C. *(DiPalma, 4/e, pp 275–286. Gilman, 8/e, pp 387–388, 396–397, 411.)* There are several chemical classes of compounds useful as antipsychotic agents. Phenothiazine derivatives (e.g., perphenazine) constitute the most numerous group and were the first antipsychotic drugs to be used. Thiothixene hydrochloride and chlorprothixene (Taractan) are two thiothixene derivatives used as antipsychotic drugs; butyrophenone derivatives are exemplified by haloperidol. Several other classes of heterocyclic compounds have antipsychotic activity, including loxapine succinate, molindone hydrochloride (Moban), and pimozide (Orap). Fluoxetine hydrochloride is used as an antidepressant; it has no significant antipsychotic activity.

252. The answer is C. *(DiPalma, 4/e, pp 244–248. Katzung, 6/e, pp 343–345.)* Triazolam is a benzodiazepine derivative, and like flurazepam and temazepam it is useful in the treatment of insomnia. It acts by binding to benzodiazepine receptors, enhancing GABA-mediated chloride influx. Adverse reactions include drowsiness, dizziness, lethargy, and ataxia. Though benzodiazepines alone do not significantly depress respiration, in combination with ethanol they can lead to severe respiratory depression. Unlike the barbiturates, benzodiazepines do not significantly induce the drug-metabolizing microsomal system at therapeutic doses.

253. The answer is D. *(DiPalma, 4/e, pp 365–374. Katzung, 6/e, pp 220–221.)* Lidocaine is an amide-type local anesthetic. It acts by interfering with influx of sodium into nerve fibers. Lidocaine is biotransformed in the liver; being an amide, it is not hydrolyzed by plasma esterases. Coadministration of epinephrine causes local vasoconstriction, thus prolonging the duration of action. Adverse reactions caused by plasma buildup include CNS excitation followed by depression and cardiovascular depression.

254. The answer is C. *(DiPalma, 4/e, pp 247–248. Gilman, 8/e, pp 424–429.)* Some benzodiazepines are biotransformed to active products with CNS effects, some of which are long-lived. Desmethyldiazepam is a long-acting metabolite of chlordiazepoxide, clorazepate, alprazolam, diazepam, and prazepam. These compounds are more likely to produce cumulative effects and residual effects such as excessive drowsiness. Oxazepam and lorazepam are biotransformed to the inactive glucuronide.

255. The answer is C. *(DiPalma, 4/e, pp 280–282. Gilman, 8/e, pp 383–401.)* The phenothiazines (e.g., thioridazine) are antipsychotic agents. Autonomic manifestations result from alpha-adrenergic receptor and muscarinic cholinergic receptor blockade. A Parkinson-like syndrome results from blockade of dopaminergic receptors in the basal ganglia. Thioridazine has a lower incidence of acute extrapyramidal reactions than higher potency agents such as haloperidol and trifluoperazine. Chronic use of all these agents often leads to tardive dyskinesia. Although effective against vomiting produced by some drugs and disease states, phenothiazines are not effective for control of motion sickness. The phenothiazines block dopaminergic receptors in the pituitary, which subsequently increases secretion of prolactin, causing hyperprolactinemia and galactorrhea.

256. The answer is D. *(DiPalma, 4/e, pp 238–239. Gilman, 8/e, pp 354–357.)* Estazolam, flurazepam, quazepam, temazepam, and triazolam are all benzodiazepine derivatives that are used exclusively for their hypnotic effect. Flurazepam can cause physical dependence but does not have analgesic properties. It undergoes an *N*-dealkylation reaction to yield *N*-desalkylflurazepam, which has an elimination half-life of 76 to 160 h.

257. The answer is E. *(DiPalma, 4/e, pp 331–332. Gilman, 8/e, pp 495–496.)* The extent and rate at which tolerance develops to the effects of opioid analgesics vary. A high degree of tolerance develops to analgesia, euphoria, sedation, respiratory depression, antidiuresis, nausea and vomiting, and cough suppression. A moderate degree develops to bradycardia. Little or no tolerance develops to the drug-induced miosis, constipation, and convulsions.

258. The answer is C. *(DiPalma, 4/e, pp 337–338. Gilman, 8/e, pp 497, 504–506.)* Methadone is an opioid receptor agonist. It is used as an analgesic and to treat opioid abstinence and heroin users (methadone maintenance). The drug has greater oral efficacy than morphine and a much longer biologic half-life; this accounts for the milder but more protracted abstinence syndrome associated with methadone. Methadone does not possess opioid antagonist properties and thus would not precipitate withdrawal symptoms in a heroin addict, as would naloxone or naltrexone.

259. The answer is D. *(DiPalma, 4/e, pp 268–269. Gilman, 8/e, pp 189–190.)* Amphetamine is a noncatechol sympathomimetic amine that is a powerful CNS stimulant and can produce psychosis and hyperthermia. It is useful in the treatment of narcolepsy. In addition to its CNS stimulatory effects, the drug has peripheral sympathomimetic properties, leading to tachycardia, cardiac arrhythmias, anginal pain, and hypertension. Amphetamine is a mixed-acting agent that (1) stimulates release of norepinephrine, (2) inhibits monoamine oxidase, and (3) produces direct receptor stimulation. The methyl group on the alpha carbon makes the compound resistant to inactivation by monoamine oxidase. Since the phenyl ring does not contain hydroxyl groups in the 3,4 positions, amphetamine is not a catechol and, therefore, not metabolized by catechol-*O*-methyltransferase (COMT).

260. The answer is C. *(DiPalma, 4/e, pp 293–297. Katzung, 6/e, p 452.)* Desipramine is a tricyclic antidepressant that acts primarily by inhibiting uptake of norepinephrine. Tricyclic antidepressants can produce many adverse reactions, including anticholinergic effects (e.g., xerostomia and constipation), sedation, orthostatic hypotension (partially owing to alpha-adrenergic blockade), tachycardia, and a decrease in REM sleep. Tricyclics also reduce the seizure threshold and can increase the risk of tonic-clonic seizures; they do not have anticonvulsant properties.

261. The answer is B. *(DiPalma, 4/e, pp 228–229. Gilman, 8/e, pp 301–303.)* Thiopental is an intravenous general anesthetic. It is very useful for short procedures because it produces a rapid recovery, which is due to redistribution out of the brain. It produces little postanesthetic excitement or vomiting. Thiopental is biotransformed in the liver by desulfuration to pentobarbital. The compound can produce cough, laryngospasm, and bronchospasm. Thiopental, unlike halothane and related inhalation anesthetics, does *not* sensitize the myocardium to endogenous catecholamines.

262. The answer is B. *(DiPalma, 4/e, pp 253–259. Gilman, 8/e, pp 370–379.)* Ethanol is a central nervous system depressant. Among its many effects, it suppresses the release of antidiuretic hormone. Ethanol also causes peripheral vasodilation, particularly of cutaneous blood vessels. Though this may give one a feeling of warmth, heat is being dissipated and body temperature is lowered. Chronic use can lead to gastritis, pancreatitis, cirrhosis of the liver, and central effects such as Wernicke's encephalopathy and Korsakoff's psychosis. Acute overdose can lead to acidosis, hypoglycemia, and elevated intracranial pressure.

263. The answer is C. *(DiPalma, 4/e, pp 291–293. Gilman, 8/e, pp 405–414.)* Amitriptyline produces a high degree of central nervous system depression and has marked anticholinergic effects. Its mechanism of action is based on its ability to inhibit the reuptake of *both* norepinephrine and serotonin in presynaptic nerve endings (in contrast to newer antidepressants like fluoxetine that block uptake of only serotonin). Cardiovascular effects include orthostatic hypotension and conduction disturbances.

264. The answer is B. *(DiPalma, 4/e, pp 365–374. Gilman, 8/e, pp 311–318.)* Lidocaine is classified as an amide local anesthetic agent and has a rapid onset of action and excellent potency. It is a versatile agent useful in many clinical applications, such as surface anesthesia, peripheral nerve block, infiltration, and spinal and epidural anesthesia. Lidocaine may be combined with epinephrine to increase the former's duration of action. The vasoconstrictor effect of epinephrine will reduce the removal of lidocaine from its site of action. Lidocaine is biotransformed in the liver by amidases and undergoes *N*-dealkylation followed by sulfate conjugation.

265. The answer is D. *(DiPalma, 4/e, pp 245–251. Katzung, 6/e, pp 338–340.)* Clorazepate is a benzodiazepine derivative, useful primarily as an antianxiety agent. The compound is inactive and must be hydrolyzed in the stomach to its active form. It can be further biotransformed in the liver; active metabolites include desmethyldiazepam and oxazepam. The metabolites have an elimination half-life of over 50 h. Prolonged use of benzodiazepines produces psychological and sometimes physical dependence.

266. The answer is D. *(DiPalma, 4/e, pp 244–251. Katzung, 6/e, pp 339–341.)* Indications for the benzodiazepines include anxiety and insomnia. Many, including chlordiazepoxide and diazepam, are used for anxiety. Flurazepam, temazepam, and triazolam are useful in the treatment of sleep disorders. Selected benzodiazepines are used in treatment of alcohol withdrawal (diazepam), seizure disorders (diazepam, clorazepate), nocturnal myoclonus (clonazepam), and skeletal muscle spasticity (diazepam). Lorazepam is useful intravenously as a premedication for endoscopic procedures or cardioversion. Chlordiazepoxide is classified as one of the long-acting benzodiazepines along with diazepam, prazepam, and clorazepate.

267. The answer is C. *(DiPalma, 4/e, pp 306–309. Gilman, 8/e, pp 439–443.)* Phenytoin's mechanism of action is based on curtailing the capacity of neurons to fire at very high frequencies. Plasma protein binding is approximately 90 percent in patients with normal amounts of circulating plasma proteins. The major clinical use is in the treatment of tonic-clonic seizures that are or become generalized complex partial seizures. The drug is not useful in absence seizures. The most common dose-related toxicity is a motor disturbance such as ataxia. Although rare, hyperplasia of the gums may occur.

268. The answer is A. *(DiPalma, 4/e, pp 286–288. Gilman, 8/e, pp 418–422.)* Lithium salts, such as lithium carbonate and lithium citrate, help to prevent the mania and to control mood swings in manic-depressive disorders. Unlike the phenothiazine derivatives, lithium is not a sedative; tremor is one of the most frequent adverse effects of lithium treatment. Renal toxicity includes lithium-induced nephrogenic diabetes insipidus and chronic interstitial nephritis during long-term therapy. Lithium also reduces thyroid function and produces edema. However, the use of diuretics to treat the lithium-induced edema will reduce the Na^+ concentrations in the body, which will promote the retention of lithium, thus increasing the potential toxicity of the drug. Since the safe and effective plasma concentration is considered to be between 0.75 and 1.25 meq/L, and concentrations above 2 meq/L have been associated with increased risk of more severe toxicity, the plasma concentrations of lithium should be monitored regularly.

269. The answer is E. *(DiPalma, 4/e, pp 244–245, 254–256. Gilman, 8/e, pp 256–257.)* GABA is an inhibitory neurotransmitter that activates the chloride channel. Benzodiazepines, e.g., chlordiazepoxide and halazepam, bind to receptors on the chloride channel and enhance the binding of GABA to its receptor. Barbiturates also act on the chloride channel to increase the frequency of opening of the channel. Valproic acid elevates brain levels of GABA by inhibiting GABA metabolism. Chlorpromazine blocks the activity of dopamine receptors and has little or no effect on the GABA system.

270. The answer is E. *(DiPalma, 4/e, pp 250–253, 270–274. Gilman, 8/e, pp 550–551.)* The active ingredient in marijuana is Δ^9-tetrahydrocannabinol. In general, marijuana is a CNS stimulant causing tachycardia, giddiness, and, at high doses, visual hallucinations. Acute intoxication is characterized by reddening of the conjunctiva (bloodshot eyes) owing to local vasodilation. Potential therapeutic uses include antiemesis in cancer chemotherapy and reduction of intraocular pressure in glaucoma. Chronic use has been associated with an "amotivational syndrome" and with a reduction in serum testosterone and sperm count. Flashbacks are a major symptom of use of lysergic acid diethylamide (LSD).

271. The answer is D. *(DiPalma, 4/e, pp 375–384. Gilman, 8/e, pp 366, 531–539.)* Physical dependence occurs following prolonged use of morphine, ethanol, barbiturates, and nonbarbiturates such as glutethimide. Acute withdrawal of these substances produces an abstinence syndrome, the severity of which depends upon the drug. Withdrawal of cocaine after chronic use can lead to craving for the drug, prolonged sleep, general fatigue, lassitude, hyperphagia, and depression. This meets the criteria for a withdrawal syndrome.

272. The answer is D. *(DiPalma, 4/e, pp 324, 342–343. Gilman, 8/e, p 488.)* Naltrexone and naloxone are pure opioid antagonists with no agonist activity at therapeutic doses. In opioid-dependent persons, these agents will precipitate withdrawal syndrome. Naltrexone is much better absorbed from the gastrointestinal tract and is useful by oral administration. It also has a much longer duration of action, making it useful in treatment programs for drug addicts. Although naltrexone does have a "first-pass" effect in the liver, the metabolic product is also active.

273. The answer is C. *(DiPalma, 4/e, pp 345–363. Gilman, 8/e, pp 656–659.)* All the drugs mentioned with the exception of acetaminophen achieve their therapeutic and toxic effects by inhibition of prostaglandin synthesis. The group includes salicylates as well as sulindac and fenoprofen and is known as nonsteroidal anti-inflammatory drugs (NSAIDS). Acetaminophen is equal in analgesic potency to NSAIDS but has no effect on prostaglandins. It is also nonulcerogenic—a great advantage in patients who are ulcer-prone.

274. The answer is B. *(DiPalma, 4/e, pp 257–258. Gilman, 8/e, pp 376, 526.)* Chronic consumption of ethanol causes hypertrophy of the hepatic smooth endoplasmic reticulum with a resultant increase in metabolic enzymes. The induction of the microsomal system may play a role in the enhanced biotransformation of ethanol and, thus, the development of metabolic or dispositional tolerance. Barbiturates are biotransformed via the microsomal system; however, in the presence of ethanol, which is preferentially metabolized, barbiturates remain active longer. Symptoms of ethanol withdrawal can include restlessness, insomnia, tremors, disorientation, hallucinations, and convulsions. Chronic effects of ethanol abuse may include gastritis, pancreatitis, hepatitis, cirrhosis of the liver, and cardiomegaly.

275. The answer is B. *(DiPalma, 4/e, pp 233–238. Gilman, 8/e, pp 358–364.)* The termination of the action of ultra-short-acting barbiturates such as methohexital and thiopental is due to redistribution of the drugs from the brain. Following redistribution thiopental is biotransformed to pentobarbital, which is further oxidized to inactive products. Chronic administration of barbiturates can induce enzymes in the liver. Barbiturates are contraindicated in acute intermittent porphyria because they increase δ-aminolevulinic acid, which produces an elevation of porphyrins in the body. In patients with acute intermittent porphyria, the precipitous increase of porphyrins may result in paralysis and death. All barbiturates possess anticonvulsant activity, but only phenobarbital, mephobarbital, and metharbital have antiepileptic properties. These drugs may be used in the treatment of tonic-clonic seizures, psychomotor seizures, and other types of epilepsy. Although alkalinization of the urine may promote the excretion of weak acidic drugs such as the barbiturates, it appears that only the excretion of phenobarbital is enhanced by increasing the pH of the urine. In the renal tubular fluid phenobarbital is converted more to the anionic form, and this form of phenobarbital is not readily reabsorbed by the renal tubular cells.

276. The answer is B. *(DiPalma, 4/e, pp 230–231. Gilman, 8/e, pp 508–517.)* The synthetic opioid fentanyl is 80 to 100 times more potent than morphine and has a major use in anesthesia. It is combined with droperidol, an antipsychotic butyrophenone, to produce neuroleptanalgesia. Muscular rigidity produced by fentanyl very likely results from opioid influence on dopaminergic transmission in the striatum, an influence that is antagonized by naloxone. Fentanyl is only available as an injection to be used intravenously in anesthesia.

277. The answer is B. *(DiPalma, 4/e, pp 220, 224–226. Gilman, 8/e, pp 286–292.)* The high solubility of halothane, a halogenated alkane, in blood and fat allows for the maintenance of anesthetic blood levels for prolonged periods. The death rate associated with halothane is similar to or slightly lower than that of other anesthetic agents. Halothane is a very potent anesthetic (MAC = 0.77) compared with nitrous oxide (MAC = 110). Hepatotoxicity does occasionally occur and appears to increase in incidence with increased exposure to halothane. Depression of respiratory centers expressed as a decreased ventilatory response to carbon dioxide occurs as anesthetic depth increases. Arterial hypotension and a reduction in cardiac output, peripheral resistance, and myocardial contractility occur at surgical levels of anesthesia.

278. The answer is E. *(DiPalma, 4/e, pp 314–318. Gilman, 8/e, pp 466–475.)* Drugs useful in the therapy of parkinsonism act through several mechanisms. Levodopa, primary therapy for parkinsonism, is the immediate precursor to dopamine and thus increases brain levels of dopamine by enhancing its synthesis. Benztropine is one of several muscarinic blocking agents and is a useful adjunct in therapy. Amantadine, an antiviral agent, acts by stimulating release of dopamine from storage sites. Bromocriptine is a direct agonist at dopaminergic receptors. Selegiline, a relatively new drug, selectively inhibits monoamine oxidase B, which is present in the brain. Monoamine oxidase A is located mainly in the liver and the gut.

279. The answer is D. *(DiPalma, 4/e, pp 325–327. Katzung, 6/e, pp 469–470.)* Codeine is an opioid analgesic useful in relieving mild-to-moderate pain. Its effects are qualitatively similar to those of morphine, but it is a less potent analgesic. It is also useful by oral administration as an antitussive agent. Adverse reactions to codeine include (1) respiratory depression, which is reversed by naloxone; (2) hypotension, cutaneous vasodilation, and urticaria, which are a result of histamine release; and (3) constipation. Codeine is biotransformed in the liver, partially by demethylation to morphine. Codeine is as addictive as other opiates and is under control of the Drug Enforcement Administration (DEA).

280. The answer is D. *(DiPalma, 4/e, pp 341–343. Gilman, 8/e, p 488.)* Naloxone is a pure opioid antagonist at μ, κ, and σ receptors. It will reverse the analgesic and other opioid effects of agonists (e.g., morphine) and agonist-antagonists (e.g., butorphanol). Naloxone will also induce withdrawal in an opioid (heroin) addict. Though naloxone will reverse opioid-induced respiratory depression, it is not effective in reversing phenobarbital-induced respiratory depression. The drug is only useful by injection for emergency treatment of opioid overdose. Naltrexone, another opioid antagonist, is useful orally for treatment of drug addiction.

281–283. The answers are 281-E, 282-K, 283-I. *(DiPalma, 4/e, pp 275–302, 312–313. Gilman, 8/e, pp 396–397.)* Amitriptyline is one of the oldest of the tricyclic antidepressants. Both amitriptyline and doxepin (Sinequan) are quite sedating and have the greatest anticholinergic activity of all the many tricyclic antidepressants available. Biotransformation by *N*-demethylation results in the production of the active metabolite, nortriptyline (which is also available for use in treatment of depression as Aventyl).

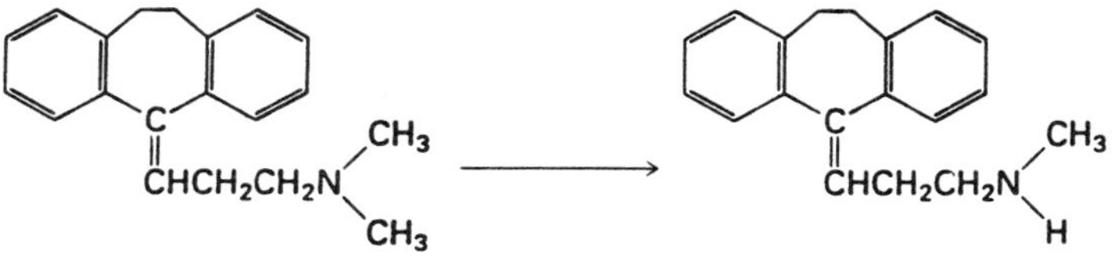

Amitriptyline Nortriptyline

Fluphenazine enanthate and fluphenazine decanoate are available for use as depot injections; these preparations have a duration of action of 1 to 4 weeks and are useful for patients with a history of poor compliance, or those with an inadequate absorption of oral medications. Haloperidol, as the decanoate salt (Haldol Decanoate), is also available for depot intramuscular injection and is usually given once every 3 to 4 weeks.

Clozapine is a low-potency drug that appears to be beneficial for use in severely ill patients who have failed to respond adequately to other antipsychotic agents. The pharmacology of this compound is atypical as compared with other antipsychotics in that it has weak dopaminergic potency, but it may alter dopaminergic function at higher centers in the brain than do other drugs. The incidence of extrapyramidal reactions (i.e., Parkinson-like symptoms and tardive dyskinesia) and elevation of prolactin concentrations are minimal. However, the most severe toxicity is the rather high incidence of agranulocytosis (approximately 1 percent); this requires that patients have regular (weekly is recommended) white blood cell counts.

284–286. The answers are 284-G, 285-L, 286-C. *(DiPalma, 4/e, pp 244–251, 268–269, 303–314. Gilman, 8/e, pp 211–212, 441–442.)*

Phenytoin is one of the most commonly used antiepileptic agents. Chronic administration has been reported to cause such adverse reactions as ataxia, dizziness, nystagmus, gingival hyperplasia, hirsutism, and megaloblastic anemia.

Diazepam is a benzodiazepine derivative and is effective in management of anxiety, as a preanesthetic medication, in alcohol withdrawal, as a skeletal muscle relaxant, and in seizure disorders. It is useful in status epilepticus, which may occur on withdrawal from a barbiturate. The agent is well absorbed orally, is highly protein-bound (greater than 90 percent), and is biotransformed in the liver to active products. Flurazepam and triazolam are benzodiazepine derivatives that are used exclusively as hypnotics.

Dextroamphetamine, a mixed-acting adrenergic drug, is more potent than the *l* isomer in producing CNS stimulation. Some central nervous system effects of use of dextroamphetamine may be increased alertness, elevated mood states, insomnia, irritability, dizziness, violent behavior, and hallucination. Although phenylephrine is an adrenergic agonist, its central stimulatory effects are minimal.

287–289. The answers are 287-D, 288-D, 289-G. *(DiPalma, 4/e, pp 233–238, 275–284, 376–378, 381–382. Katzung, 6/e, pp 469–473.)* Heroin and other opioids (such as morphine and meperidine) exhibit a high degree of tolerance and physical dependence. The magnitudes of rates of tolerance to all the effects of opioids are not necessarily the same. The physical dependence is quite clear from the character and severity of withdrawal symptoms, which include vomiting spasms, abdominal cramps, diarrhea, and acid-base imbalances among others.

Secobarbital exhibits the same pharmacologic properties as other members of the barbiturate class. While there may be considerable tolerance to the sedative and intoxicating effects of the drug, the lethal dose is not much greater in addicted than normal persons. Severe withdrawal symptoms in epileptic patients may include grand mal seizures and delirium.

No current evidence exists that chlorpromazine, an antipsychotic agent, is addicting. Although some tolerance and physical dependence have been suggested, the failure to detect any EEG changes upon abrupt cessation of the drug implies that these effects are not of major importance.

None of these drugs have significant association with hallucinations or psychedelic effects. Lysergic acid diethylamide (LSD) is the primary agent deemed to possess these attributes.

Autonomic Nervous System

General Considerations
- Anatomic
- Physiologic
- Nature of synaptic transmission
- Cholinergic transmission
- Adrenergic transmission
- Receptors, adrenergic and cholinergic

Adrenergic Drugs
- Sites and mode of action
- Chemistry and structure-activity relationships
- Direct-acting agonists
  - Epinephrine*
  - Norepinephrine*
  - Isoproterenol*
  - Phenylephrine
  - Dobutamine
  - Salmeterol
  - Terbutaline
  - Albuterol*
  - Pirbuterol
  - Bitolterol
  - Metaproterenol
  - Isoetharine
  - Ritodrine
  - Tetrahydrozoline
- Indirect-acting agents
  - Tyramine*
- Mixed-acting agents
  - Dopamine*
  - Ephedrine*
  - Phenylpropanolamine
  - Amphetamines
  - Pseudoephedrine
  - Metaraminol

Beta-Adrenergic Blocking Drugs
- Propranolol*
- Acebutolol
- Atenolol
- Betaxolol
- Bisoprolol
- Carteolol
- Esmolol
- Labetalol
- Metoprolol
- Nadolol
- Penbutolol
- Pindolol
- Sotalol
- Timolol

Alpha-Adrenergic Blocking Drugs
- Nonselective
  - Phentolamine*
  - Phenoxybenzamine*
- Selective
  - Prazosin,* terazosin, doxazosin
  - Yohimbine

Adrenergic Neuronal Blocking Drugs
- Reserpine*
- Guanethidine,* guanadrel
- Metyrosine

Cholinomimetic Agents
- Direct-acting
  - Choline esters
    - Acetylcholine*

- Methacholine
- Carbachol
- Bethanechol
- Naturally occurring muscarinic alkaloids
  - Muscarine*
  - Pilocarpine*
- Naturally occurring nicotinic alkaloids
  - Nicotine*
  - Lobeline

Indirect Acting

- Reversible cholinesterase inhibitors
  - Physostigmine*
  - Neostigmine
  - Pyridostigmine
  - Edrophonium
  - Ambenonium chloride
  - Tacrine
- Irreversible cholinesterase inhibitors
  - Isoflurophate*
  - Echothiophate iodide
  - Malathion*
  - Soman, sarin, tabun

Antidotes for Organophosphate Poisoning

- Atropine
- Pralidoxime chloride

Antimuscarinic Drugs

- Atropine*
- Homatropine*
- Scopolamine*
- Propantheline bromide
- Cyclopentolate
- Tropicamide
- Dicyclomine
- Ipratropium
- Methscopolamine
- Trihexyphenidyl*

Ganglionic Blocking Drugs

- Mecamylamine
- Trimethaphan camsylate
- Nicotine

Skeletal-Muscle Relaxants

- Neuromuscular blocking agents
  - Depolarizing drugs
    - Succinylcholine*
  - Nondepolarizing drugs
    - Tubocurarine*
    - Metocurine
    - Gallamine
    - Doxacurium
    - Mivacurium
    - Pipecuronium
    - Pancuronium
    - Vecuronium
    - Atracurium
- Centrally acting skeletal-muscle relaxants
  - Baclofen
  - Cyclobenzaprine
  - Diazepam
- Direct-acting skeletal-muscle relaxant
  - Dantrolene

MAO Inhibitors

- Selegiline*
- Tranylcypromine
- Phenelzine

DIRECTIONS: Each question below contains five suggested responses. Select the **one best** response to each question.

290. Of the many types of adrenergic receptors found throughout the body, which is most likely responsible for the cardiac stimulation observed following an intravenous injection of epinephrine?

(A) $Alpha_1$-adrenergic receptors
(B) $Alpha_2$-adrenergic receptors
(C) $Beta_1$-adrenergic receptors
(D) $Beta_2$-adrenergic receptors
(E) $Beta_3$-adrenergic receptors

291. The enzyme that is inhibited by echothiophate iodide (Phospholine Iodide) is

(A) tyrosine hydroxylase
(B) acetylcholinesterase
(C) catechol-*O*-methyltransferase
(D) monoamine oxidase
(E) carbonic anhydrase

292. Applied to the skin in a transdermal patch (transdermal therapeutic delivery system), this drug is used to prevent or reduce the occurrence of nausea and vomiting associated with motion sickness.

(A) Diphenhydramine
(B) Chlorpromazine
(C) Ondansetron
(D) Dimenhydrinate
(E) Scopolamine

293. The nonselective beta-adrenergic blocking agent that is also a competitive antagonist at $alpha_1$-adrenoceptors is

(A) timolol (Blocadren)
(B) nadolol (Corgard)
(C) pindolol (Visken)
(D) acebutolol (Sectral)
(E) labetalol (Normodyne)

294. The contractile effect of various doses of norepinephrine (X) alone on vascular smooth muscle is represented in the figure below.

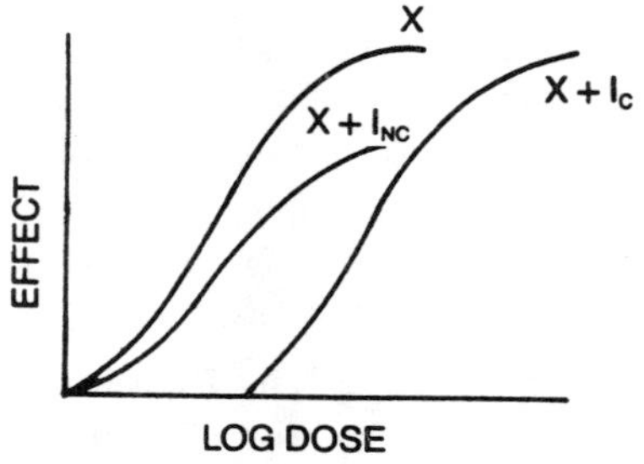

When combined with an antagonist (I_C or I_{NC}), a shift in the dose-response curve occurs. The curve labeled X + I_{NC} would most likely occur when vascular smooth muscle is treated with norepinephrine in the presence of

(A) terazosin
(B) phentolamine
(C) labetalol
(D) phenoxybenzamine
(E) prazosin

---

295. The reversible cholinesterase inhibitor indicated in the treatment of Alzheimer's disease is

(A) tacrine
(B) edrophonium
(C) neostigmine
(D) pyridostigmine
(E) ambenonium

296. Hypotension, bradycardia, respiratory depression, and muscle weakness, all unresponsive to atropine and neostigmine, would most likely be due to

(A) diazoxide
(B) isoflurophate
(C) tubocurarine
(D) nicotine
(E) pilocarpine

297. Ritodrine hydrochloride (Yutopar) is used in the treatment of

(A) Parkinson's disease
(B) bronchial asthma
(C) depression
(D) hypertension
(E) premature labor

298. The skeletal muscle relaxant that acts directly on the contractile mechanism of the muscle fibers is

(A) gallamine (Flaxedil)
(B) baclofen (Lioresal)
(C) pancuronium (Pavulon)
(D) cyclobenzaprine (Flexeril)
(E) dantrolene (Dantrium)

299. A predictably dangerous side effect of nadolol (Corgard) that constitutes a contraindication to its clinical use in susceptible patients is the induction of

(A) hypertension
(B) cardiac arrhythmia
(C) asthmatic attacks
(D) respiratory depression
(E) hypersensitivity

300. All the following drugs are used topically in the treatment of chronic wide-angle glaucoma. Which of these agents reduces intraocular pressure by decreasing the formation of the aqueous humor?

(A) Betaxolol hydrochloride (Betoptic)
(B) Echothiophate iodide (Phospholine Iodide)
(C) Pilocarpine hydrochloride (Pilocar)
(D) Isoflurophate (Floropryl)
(E) Physostigmine salicylate (Isopto Eserine)

301. The cholinomimetic drug that is useful for treating postoperative abdominal distention and gastric atony is

(A) acetylcholine (Miochol)
(B) methacholine (Provocholine)
(C) carbachol (Isopto Carbachol)
(D) bethanechol (Urecholine)
(E) pilocarpine (Pilocar)

302. Neostigmine (Prostigmin) will effectively antagonize skeletal muscle relaxation produced by

(A) metocurine (Metubine)
(B) succinylcholine (Anectine)
(C) diazepam (Valium)
(D) baclofen (Lioresal)
(E) nicotine (Nicorette)

303. Which of the following bronchodilators is the most selective $beta_2$-adrenergic agonist, is long-acting, and can be administered by oral inhalation?

(A) Salmeterol (Serevent)
(B) Terbutaline (Brethine)
(C) Pirbuterol (Maxair)
(D) Metaproterenol (Alupent)
(E) Isoetharine (Bronkosol)

304. Pralidoxime chloride (Protopam Chloride) is a drug that

(A) reduces the vesicular stores of catecholamines in adrenergic and dopaminergic neurons
(B) blocks the active transport of choline into cholinergic neurons
(C) reactivates cholinesterases that have been inhibited by organophosphate cholinesterase inhibitors
(D) stimulates the activity of phospholipase C with increased formation of inositol triphosphate
(E) inhibits the reuptake of biogenic amines into nerve terminals

305. Which of the following antimuscarinic drugs is used by inhalation in the treatment of bronchial asthma?

(A) Dicyclomine hydrochloride (Bentyl)
(B) Cyclopentolate hydrochloride (Cyclogyl)
(C) Ipratropium bromide (Atrovent)
(D) Methscopolamine bromide (Pamine)
(E) Trihexyphenidyl hydrochloride (Artane)

306. The cholinesterase inhibitor that is used in the diagnosis of myasthenia gravis is

(A) edrophonium chloride (Tensilon)
(B) ambenonium chloride (Mytelase)
(C) malathion (Ovide)
(D) physostigmine salicylate (Antilirium)
(E) pyridostigmine bromide (Mestinon)

307. Epinephrine may be mixed with certain anesthetics, such as procaine, in order to

(A) stimulate local wound repair
(B) promote hemostasis
(C) enhance their interaction with neural membranes and their ability to depress nerve conduction
(D) retard their systemic absorption
(E) facilitate their distribution along nerves and fascial planes

308. The skeletal muscles that are most sensitive to the action of tubocurarine are the

(A) muscles of the trunk
(B) muscles of the arms and legs
(C) respiratory muscles
(D) muscles of the head, neck, and face
(E) abdominal muscles

309. The drug of choice for the treatment of anaphylactic shock is

(A) epinephrine
(B) norepinephrine
(C) isoproterenol
(D) diphenhydramine
(E) atropine

310. Both phentolamine (Regitine) and prazosin (Minipress)

(A) are competitive antagonists at $alpha_1$-adrenergic receptors
(B) have potent direct vasodilator actions on vascular smooth muscle
(C) enhance gastric acid secretion via a histamine-like effect
(D) cause hypotension and bradycardia
(E) are used chronically for the treatment of primary hypertension

311. Pancuronium bromide (Pavulon) may cause an increased heart rate due to

(A) a reflex response to hypotension caused by the drug
(B) blockade of N_N receptors in parasympathetic ganglia
(C) its vagolytic action on the heart
(D) a digitalis-like action on the myocardium
(E) direct stimulation of the vasomotor center in the brainstem

DIRECTIONS: Each numbered question or incomplete statement below is NEGATIVELY phrased. Select the **one best** lettered response.

312. All the following are possible effects of low doses of nicotine (from smoking tobacco products) EXCEPT

(A) increased tone and motor activity of the intestine
(B) stimulation of respiratory rate and depth
(C) stimulation of catecholamine release from the adrenal medulla
(D) bradycardia
(E) nausea and vomiting

313. All the following drugs have significant antimuscarinic effects EXCEPT

(A) diphenhydramine (Benadryl)
(B) pyridostigmine (Mestinon)
(C) meperidine (Demerol)
(D) amitriptyline (Elavil)
(E) thioridazine (Mellaril)

314. All the following neuromuscular blocking agents are biotransformed by either deacetylation or ester hydrolysis, which results in the formation of an active skeletal muscle relaxant, EXCEPT

(A) atracurium besylate (Tracrium)
(B) pancuronium bromide (Pavulon)
(C) pipecuronium bromide (Arduan)
(D) succinylcholine chloride (Anectine)
(E) vecuronium bromide (Norcuron)

315. All the following statements are true concerning isoproterenol (Isuprel) EXCEPT that

(A) it is readily absorbed when administered parenterally or by aerosol
(B) it lowers peripheral resistance and diastolic blood pressure
(C) it relaxes bronchial smooth muscle
(D) it is biotransformed primarily in the liver by monoamine oxidase (MAO)
(E) it is used as a cardiac stimulant in heart block and cardiogenic shock after myocardial infarction

316. Propranolol (Inderal) is either contraindicated in, or should be used with caution in, all the following disease states EXCEPT

(A) hypoglycemia
(B) Raynaud's phenomenon
(C) bronchial asthma
(D) congestive heart failure
(E) angina pectoris

317. All the following structures respond to beta-adrenergic receptor stimulation EXCEPT

(A) the ciliary muscle of the iris
(B) the radial muscle of the iris
(C) bronchial muscle
(D) the atrioventricular node
(E) the sinoatrial node

318. All the following drugs act within sympathetic neurons to depress neurotransmitter release and are used to treat hypertension EXCEPT

(A) guanadrel (Hylorel)
(B) metyrosine (Demser)
(C) selegiline (Eldepryl)
(D) reserpine (Serpasil)
(E) guanethidine (Ismelin)

319. All the following statements are true concerning the use of dopamine (Intropin) EXCEPT

(A) this drug must be given by intravenous infusion since it is rapidly biotransformed
(B) small doses of dopamine cause an increase in glomerular filtration rate, renal blood flow, and Na^+ excretion
(C) at intermediate concentrations, the administration of dopamine results in a positive inotropic effect on the myocardium
(D) high concentrations of dopamine cause vasoconstriction, increased peripheral vascular resistance, and elevation of mean blood pressure
(E) central nervous system adverse effects (including sedation, lethargy, and depression) are commonly experienced by patients during the administration of the drug

320. Atropine and scopolamine will block all the effects of acetylcholine listed below EXCEPT

(A) bradycardia
(B) salivary secretion
(C) bronchoconstriction
(D) skeletal muscle contraction
(E) miosis

321. All the following statements are true for both terbutaline (Brethine) and isoetharine (Bronkosol) EXCEPT

(A) these drugs are direct-acting, selective $beta_2$-adrenergic receptor agonists
(B) both compounds will increase adenylate cyclase activity in bronchiolar smooth muscle
(C) extensive first-pass biotransformation of these drugs will occur following oral administration
(D) both compounds can be given by inhalation or orally for the treatment of bronchospasm
(E) two common adverse effects associated with these drugs are muscle tremors and tachycardia

322. Propranolol (Inderal) is indicated for use in patients with all the following conditions EXCEPT

(A) hypertension
(B) angina pectoris
(C) glaucoma
(D) migraine headaches
(E) supraventricular and ventricular arrhythmias

323. All the following statements are true concerning the use of therapeutic oral doses of amphetamine EXCEPT

(A) the drug may cause hypotension by decreasing both systolic and diastolic blood pressure
(B) wakefulness, alertness, headache, and agitation are common CNS effects of the drug
(C) anorexia is a common effect of this drug
(D) narcolepsy and attention-deficit hyperactivity disorder are approved indications for amphetamine
(E) amphetamine induces the release of biogenic amines from storage sites in neuron terminals

324. All the following statements are accurate characterizations of ephedrine EXCEPT that it

(A) is used as a decongestant
(B) can cause insomnia, restlessness, agitation, and tremors
(C) can increase systemic blood pressure
(D) is rapidly biotransformed by both catechol-*O*-methyltransferase (COMT) and monoamine oxidase (MAO)
(E) will relax the smooth muscles of the bronchial tree

325. All the following are possible effects of mecamylamine (Inversine) EXCEPT

(A) arteriolar vasodilatation
(B) mydriasis and cycloplegia
(C) constipation and urinary retention
(D) tachycardia
(E) skeletal muscle weakness

326. All the following statements are true concerning dobutamine hydrochloride (Dobutrex) EXCEPT that it

(A) is a selective agonist at $beta_1$-adrenergic receptors
(B) activates dopaminergic receptors in renal and mesenteric vascular beds
(C) is used to increase cardiac output in patients with severe cardiac failure
(D) must be given by intravenous administration
(E) may cause tachycardia and anginal pain

327. All the following are effects elicited by activation of the parasympathetic nervous system EXCEPT

(A) decreased heart rate
(B) increased tone of longitudinal smooth muscles of the intestine
(C) contraction of skeletal muscles
(D) contraction of the detrusor of the urinary bladder
(E) secretion of fluid from the lacrimal glands

328. All the following compounds are believed to function as cotransmitters or neuromodulators that exist with acetylcholine or norepinephrine in neurons of the autonomic nervous system EXCEPT

(A) vasoactive intestinal peptide (VIP)
(B) adenosine triphosphate (ATP)
(C) neuropeptide Y (NPY)
(D) substance P
(E) serotonin (5-HT)

DIRECTIONS: Each group of questions below consists of lettered headings followed by a set of numbered items. For each numbered item, select the **one** lettered heading with which it is **most** closely associated. Each lettered heading may be used **once, more than once, or not at all.**

Questions 329–331

For each pharmacologic action listed, select the drug with which it is most likely to be associated.

(A) Diazepam (Valium)
(B) Doxazosin (Cardura)
(C) Scopolamine (Transderm Scop)
(D) Cyclobenzaprine hydrochloride (Flexeril)
(E) Propantheline bromide (Pro-Banthine)
(F) Atracurium besylate (Tracrium)
(G) Atenolol (Tenormin)
(H) Baclofen (Lioresal)
(I) Timolol maleate (Timoptic)
(J) Phentolamine mesylate (Regitine)

329. Reduces intraocular pressure

330. Causes skeletal muscle paralysis

331. Is a selective $alpha_1$-adrenergic antagonist

Questions 332–334

For each anatomic site listed, select the catecholamine neurotransmitter found in the highest amounts.

(A) Dopamine
(B) Serotonin
(C) Epinephrine
(D) Norepinephrine
(E) Acetylcholine

332. Adrenergic fibers

333. Adrenal medulla

334. Caudate nucleus

Questions 335–337

The figure below illustrates proposed sites of action of drugs. For each drug listed, select the site of action that the drug is most likely to *inhibit* (α = alpha receptor; β = beta receptor; COMT = catechol-*O*-methyltransferase; MAO = monoamine oxidase; NE = norepinephrine; NMN = normetanephrine).

SYMPATHETIC NEUROEFFECTOR JUNCTION

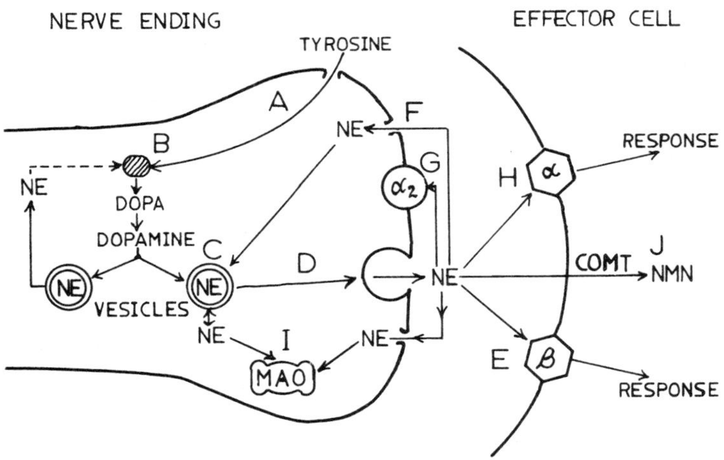

335. Reserpine

336. Esmolol

337. Tranylcypromine

Questions 338–340

For each of the naturally occurring amines below, select the appropriate structure.

A 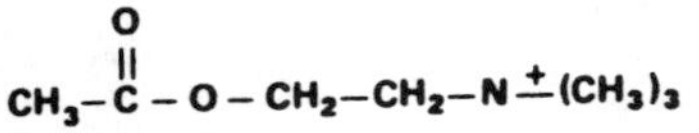

B 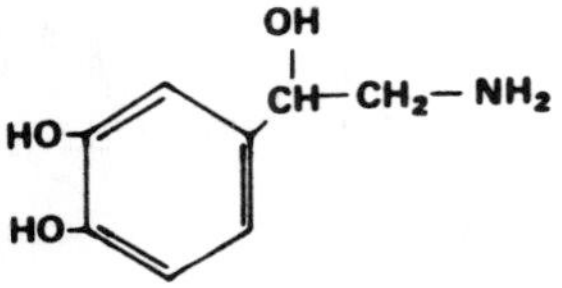

C 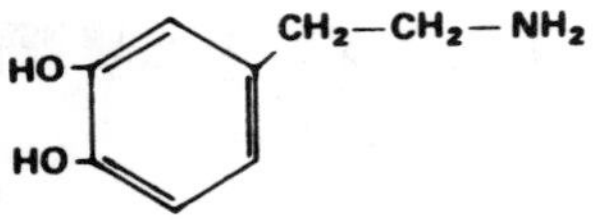

D 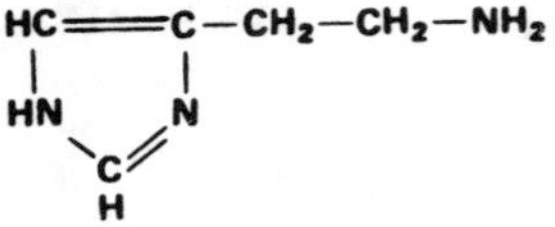

E 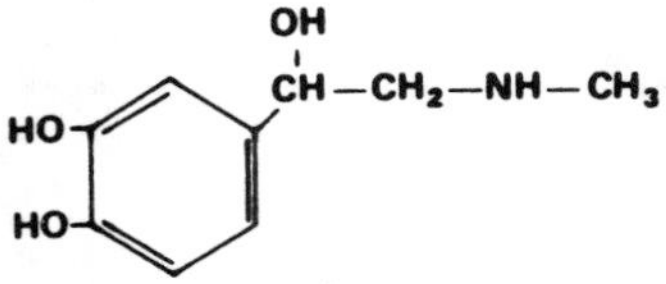

338. Acetylcholine

339. Histamine

340. Epinephrine

Questions 341–343

For each of the neurotransmitters below, select the amino acid from which it is synthesized.

(A) Tyrosine
(B) Serine
(C) Histidine
(D) Tryptophan
(E) Hydroxyproline

341. Epinephrine

342. Histamine

343. Serotonin

Questions 344–346

Match the descriptions of use with the appropriate drug.

(A) Tropicamide (Mydriacyl)
(B) Methylphenidate (Ritalin)
(C) Propantheline (Pro-Banthine)
(D) Ritodrine (Yutopar)
(E) Guanethidine (Ismelin)

344. Used as an antihypertensive drug

345. Used in the treatment of gastrointestinal hypermotility

346. Used as an adjunct in the therapy of hyperkinetic syndromes

Questions 347–349

For each of the drugs below, select its appropriate site of action in the acetylcholine system diagrammed.

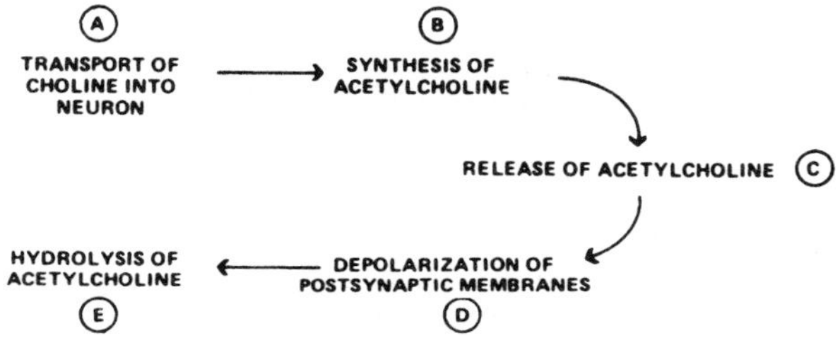

347. Botulinus toxin

348. Hemicholinium

349. Muscarine

Autonomic Nervous System

Answers

290. The answer is C. *(DiPalma, 4/e, pp 102, 110, 116–119.)* Stimulation of both the contractile and rhythmic effects of epinephrine on the heart is mediated through activation of postsynaptic beta$_1$-adrenergic receptors. These receptor sites mediate an epinephrine-induced increased firing rate of the sinoatrial (SA) node, increased conduction velocity through the atrioventricular (AV) node and the His-Purkinje system, and increased contractility and conduction velocity of atrial and ventricular muscle. Epinephrine activation of alpha-adrenoceptors does not affect cardiac function. Beta$_2$-adrenergic receptors play a minor role in cardiac stimulation. They are more important in the relaxation of tracheobronchial smooth muscle, relaxation of the detrusor of the urinary bladder, dilation of arterioles that serve skeletal muscles, and increased secretion of insulin by the pancreas. Lipolysis in fat cells and melatonin secretion by the pineal gland appear to involve stimulation of beta$_3$-adrenergic receptors.

291. The answer is B. *(AMA Drug Evaluations Annual, 1993, pp 2057, 2065. DiPalma, 4/e, pp 155, 160–161.)* Echothiophate iodide is a long-acting (irreversible) cholinesterase inhibitor. It is used topically in the eye for the treatment of various types of glaucoma. Maximum reduction of intraocular pressure occurs within 24 h and the effect may persist for several days. The drug is a water-soluble compound, which affords it a practical advantage over the lipid-soluble isoflurophate (another cholinesterase inhibitor used to treat glaucoma).

292. The answer is E. *(DiPalma, 4/e, p 168. Gilman, 8/e, pp 163–164.)* All the drugs listed in the question are used as antiemetics. Chlopromazine (Thorazine) is a general antiemetic, used orally, rectally, or by injection for the control of nausea and vomiting that is caused by conditions that are not necessarily defined. Ondansetron (Zofran) is indicated in the oral or intravenous route for the prevention of nausea and vomiting caused by cancer chemotherapy. Diphenhydramine (Benadryl) and dimenhydrinate (Dramamine) are used orally for the active and prophylactic treatment of motion sickness. Scopolamine (Transderm-Scop) is a transdermal preparation used in the prevention of motion sickness. The drug is incorporated into a bandagelike adhesive unit that is placed behind the ear. The scopolamine delivered in this manner is well absorbed and maintains an effect for up to 72 h. Other drugs that are prepared for transdermal delivery include clonidine (an antihypertensive agent), estradiol (an estrogen), fentanyl (an opioid analgesic), nicotine (a smoking deterrent), nitroglycerin (an antianginal drug), and testosterone (an androgen).

293. The answer is E. *(DiPalma, 4/e, pp 137–138. Gilman, 8/e, pp 235–236.)* With the exception of acebutolol—which is classified as a "cardioselective," or selective, $beta_1$-adrenergic blocking agent—all the listed drugs are considered to be nonselective beta-adrenergic blocking agents because they will competitively antagonize agonists at both $beta_1$- and $beta_2$-adrenergic receptor sites. Labetalol is unique in that it is, at therapeutic doses, also a competitive antagonist at $alpha_1$-adrenergic receptors. The drug has more potent blocking activity at beta-adrenoceptors; the potency ratio for alpha:beta blockade is 1:3 for the oral route and 1:7 after intravenous administration. Similar to the other beta-adrenergic blocking drugs, labetalol is indicated for the treatment of essential hypertension; however, because of the $alpha_1$-adrenergic blocking activity, blood pressure is often decreased more in the standing than in the supine position and symptoms of postural hypotension can occur.

294. The answer is D. *(DiPalma, 4/e, pp 24, 138, 139–143.)* Competitive antagonists produce a parallel shift to the right in the dose-response curve of an agonist without a reduction in the maximal effect. This type of inhibition of agonist response is due to the reversible binding of the antagonist with the affected receptor site(s); this is exemplified in the curve shown for the agonist norepinephrine (X) plus an antagonist (N_C). Noncompetitive antagonists prevent an agonist from inducing any effect at a given receptor site and thus reduce the number of receptor sites that can be stimulated by an agonist. These compounds produce a nonparallel shift in the dose-response curve of the agonist and a diminution in the maximum response, as shown by the curve labeled $X + I_{NC}$.

Norepinephrine contracts vascular smooth muscle by binding to and activating $alpha_1$-adrenergic receptors. Phentolamine, prazosin, terazosin, and labetalol all bind to $alpha_1$-adrenergic receptors, but fail to activate them. Since the action of these compounds is reversible, these drugs act as competitive antagonists of norepinephrine at these receptor sites. Phenoxybenzamine is an alkylating agent that forms a stable covalent bond with both $alpha_1$- and $alpha_2$-adrenergic receptors. This long-lasting receptor blockade cannot be overcome by competition with an agonist. Therefore, in contrast to the other drugs listed, blockade with phenoxybenzamine is not reversible, is referred to as *nonequilibrium receptor blockade*, and in the presence of an alpha-adrenergic receptor agonist such as norepinephrine will result in a dose-response curve exemplified by curve $X + I_{NC}$.

295. The answer is A. *(DiPalma, 4/e, pp 159–160. Katzung, 6/e, p 927.)* Patients with Alzheimer's disease present with progressive impairment of memory and cognitive functions such as a lack of attention, disturbed language function, and an inability to complete common tasks. Although the exact defect in the central nervous system (CNS) has not been elucidated, evidence suggests that a reduction in cholinergic nerve function is largely responsible for the symptoms.

Tacrine (tetrahydroaminoacridine) has been found to be somewhat effective in patients with mild-to-moderate symptoms of this disease for improvement of cognitive functions. The drug is primarily a reversible cholinesterase inhibitor that increases the concentration of functional acetylcholine in the brain. However, the pharmacology of tacrine is complex; the drug also acts as a muscarinic receptor modulator in that it has partial agonistic activity as well as weak antagonistic activity on muscarinic receptors in the CNS. In addition, tacrine appears to enhance the release of acetylcholine from cholinergic nerves and it may alter the concentrations of other neurotransmitters such as dopamine and norepinephrine.

Of all the reversible cholinesterase inhibitors, only tacrine and physostigmine cross the blood-brain barrier in sufficient amounts to make these compounds useful for disorders involving the CNS. Physostigmine has been tried as a therapy for Alzheimer's disease; however, it is more commonly used to antagonize the effects of toxic concentrations of drugs with antimuscarinic properties, including atropine, antihistamines, phenothiazines, and tricyclic antidepressants. Neostigmine, pyridostigmine, and ambenonium are used mainly in the treatment of myasthenia gravis; edrophonium is useful for the diagnosis of this muscular disease.

296. The answer is D. *(DiPalma, 4/e, pp 151–153. Gilman, 8/e, pp 180–181.)* Nicotine is a depolarizing ganglionic blocking agent that initially stimulates and then blocks N_N (ganglionic) and N_M (skeletal muscle) cholinergic receptors. Blockade of the sympathetic division of the autonomic nervous system results in arteriolar vasodilation, bradycardia, and hypotension. Blockade at the neuromuscular junction leads to muscle weakness and respiratory depression caused by interference with the function of the diaphragm and intercostal muscles. Atropine, a muscarinic receptor blocker, would be an effective antagonist, as would neostigmine, a cholinesterase inhibitor. Pilocarpine and isoflurophate are cholinomimetics and can be antagonized by atropine; the effects of tubocurarine can be inhibited by neostigmine. Diazoxide, a vasodilator, would cause tachycardia, rather than bradycardia.

297. The answer is E. *(AMA Drug Evaluations Annual, 1993, pp 1161–1163.)* Ritodrine hydrochloride is a selective $beta_2$-adrenergic agonist that relaxes uterine smooth muscle. It also has the other effects attributable to beta-adrenergic receptor stimulants, such as bronchodilation, cardiac stimulation, enhanced renin secretion, and hyperglycemia. Of all the selective $beta_2$-adrenergic receptor agonists available in the United States, ritodrine is the only one approved for use in premature labor, although terbutaline sulfate (Brethine) is being evaluated in clinical trials for this indication.

298. The answer is E. *(DiPalma, 4/e, p 180. Katzung, 6/e, pp 416–417.)* There are three major classes of skeletal muscle relaxants: peripherally acting, centrally acting, and direct-acting. The peripherally acting drugs include the nondepolarizing (e.g., tubocurarine, gallamine, pancuronium) and depolarizing (e.g., succinylcholine, decamethonium) neuromuscular blockers that antagonize acetylcholine at the muscle end-plate (i.e., at N_M receptors). Centrally acting skeletal muscle relaxants (e.g., diazepam, cyclobenzaprine, baclofen) interfere with transmission along the monosynaptic and polysynaptic neural pathways in the spinal cord. Dantrolene, the only direct-acting skeletal muscle relaxant, affects the excitation-contraction coupling mechanism of skeletal muscle by depressing the release of ionic calcium from the sarcoplasmic reticulum to the myoplasma. The drug is also useful in the prevention and management of malignant hyperthermia induced by general anesthetics.

299. The answer is C. *(DiPalma, 4/e, p 136. Gilman, 8/e, pp 232–233.)* The chief danger of therapy with beta-adrenergic blocking agents such as nadolol (Corgard) and propranolol (Inderal) is associated with the blockade itself. Beta-adrenergic blockade results in an increase in airway resistance that can be fatal in asthmatic patients. Hypersensitivity reactions such as rash, fever, and purpura are rare and necessitate discontinuation of therapy.

300. The answer is A. *(AMA Drug Evaluations Annual, 1993, pp 2057, 2059–2061, 2065. Gilman, 8/e, pp 143–144, 238, 240.)* When applied topically to the eye, both the direct-acting cholinomimetic agents (e.g., pilocarpine) and those cholinomimetic drugs that act by inhibition of acetylcholinesterase (e.g., echothiophate, isoflurophate, and physostigmine) cause miosis by contracting the sphincter muscle of the iris and reduction of ocular pressure by contraction of the ciliary muscle. In patients with glaucoma, this latter effect permits greater drainage of the aqueous humor through the trabecular meshwork in the canal of Schlemm and a reduction in resistance to outflow of the aqueous humor. Certain beta-adrenergic blocking agents (e.g., betaxolol, timolol, and levobunolol) applied to the eye are also very useful in treating chronic wide-angle glaucoma. These drugs appear to act by decreasing the secretion (or formation) of the aqueous humor by antagonizing the effect of circulating catecholamines on beta-adrenergic receptors in the ciliary epithelium.

301. The answer is D. *(DiPalma, 4/e, pp 149–151. Gilman, 8/e, pp 124, 126–127.)* Of the four choline esters (acetylcholine, methacholine, carbachol, and bethanechol), the latter two drugs have the greatest agonistic activity on muscarinic receptors of the gastrointestinal tract and urinary bladder. Bethanechol is used orally or by subcutaneous injection as a stimulant of the smooth muscles of the gastrointestinal tract (for cases of postoperative abdominal distention, gastric atony and retention or gastroparesis) and the urinary bladder (for nonobstructive postoperative and postpartum urinary retention). Carbachol is not used for these purposes due to significant activity at nicotinic receptors at autonomic ganglia; the drug is useful as a miotic for treating glaucoma and in certain types of ocular surgery. Acetycholine is occasionally used topically during cataract surgery; metacholine is used by inhalation for the diagnosis of bronchial hyperreactivity in patients who do not have clinically apparent asthma. Pilocarpine (a naturally occurring alkaloid) is a drug of choice for the treatment of glaucoma.

302. The answer is A. *(DiPalma, 4/e, pp 156–158. Gilman, 8/e, p 176.)* Anticholinesterase agents, such as neostigmine, will delay the catabolism of acetylcholine released from parasympathetic autonomic and somatic nerve terminals. At the neuromuscular junction this results in increased competition for the N_M receptors by acetylcholine (the agonist) and the curariform drugs (the antagonists) such as tubocurarine, metocurine, and pancuronium. In addition, neostigmine has a direct stimulating action on the skeletal muscle junction, which enhances its ability to antagonize the competitive neuromuscular blockers. The activity of succinylcholine at the neuromuscular junction will be exacerbated by neostigmine, since succinylcholine is inactivated by acetylcholinesterase. The skeletal muscle relaxation that may result from toxic doses of nicotine-blocking N_M receptors will be unaffected by neostigmine. Diazepam and baclofen are centrally acting skeletal muscle relaxants whose effects are not altered by the peripheral actions of neostigmine.

303. The answer is A. *(DiPalma, 4/e, pp 123–124. Katzung, 6/e, p 314.)* All of these drugs are selective beta$_2$-adrenergic agonists that relax bronchial smooth muscle; i.e., they stimulate bronchial beta$_2$-adrenergic receptors at lower doses than cardiac beta$_1$-adrenergic receptors. All are indicated for use in patients with bronchial asthma or reversible bronchospasm and all are available for use by inhalation through the mouth. In vitro studies have shown that salmeterol is up to 100 times more selective than terbutaline and albuterol (Ventolin, Proventil), previously the most selective beta$_2$-adrenergic agonists available for therapeutic use. Although terbutaline and albuterol are considered to be long-acting (duration of action of approximately 4 to 6 h following inhalation) in comparison to epinephrine, isoproterenol, and isoetharine (duration of action of about 1 to 3 h), salmeterol has the longest duration of action (approximately 12 h); therefore, this drug is administered only twice daily (at 12-h intervals) by oral inhalation.

304. The answer is C. *(DiPalma, 4/e, pp 160–162. Gilman, 8/e, pp 141–142.)* Organophosphate cholinesterase inhibitors react with both acetylcholinesterase and serum cholinesterase (pseudocholinesterase) by phosphorylating the enzymes, thus rendering them inactive, inasmuch as the phosphorylated enzyme hydrolyzes esters very slowly. Pralidoxime chloride (also known as 2-PAM chloride) is an oxime derivative that can cause dephosphorylation of the enzyme if it is administered within a short time after the organophosphate. If not administered promptly, the phosphorylated enzyme will lose an alkyl or alkoxy group (a process called "aging"), leaving a more stable phosphorylated enzyme that then cannot be dephosphorylated. The time period during which this occurs depends upon the nature of the phosphoryl group and the rapidity with which the organophosphate compound affects the enzyme. This can be from a few seconds to several hours.

305. The answer is C. *(Gilman, 8/e, pp 159–160, 162–163, 476.)* A wide variety of clinical conditions are treated with antimuscarinic drugs. Dicyclomine hydrochloride (Bentyl) and methscopolamine bromide (Pamine) are used to reduce gastrointestinal motility, although side effects—e.g., dryness of the mouth, loss of visual accommodation, and difficulty in urination—may limit their acceptance by patients. Cyclopentolate hydrochloride (Cyclogyl) is used in ophthalmology for its mydriatic and cycloplegic properties during refraction of the eye. Trihexyphenidyl hydrochloride (Artane) is one of the important antimuscarinic compounds used in the treatment of parkinsonism. For bronchodilation in patients with bronchial asthma and other bronchospastic diseases, ipratropium bromide (Atrovent) is used by inhalation. Systemic adverse reactions are low since the actions are largely confined to the mouth and airways.

306. The answer is A. *(AMA Drug Evaluations Annual, 1993, pp 394–398.)* Although all the listed compounds inhibit the activity of the cholinesterases, only edrophonium chloride is used in the diagnosis of myasthenia gravis. The drug has a more rapid onset of action (1 to 3 min following intravenous administration) and a shorter duration of action (approximately 5 to 10 min) than pyridostigmine bromide and ambenonium chloride. It is more water-soluble than physostigmine salicylate and, therefore, produces no clinically significant adverse effects on the CNS. Pyridostigmine bromide and ambenonium chloride are used in the treatment of this muscle weakness disease. Physostigmine salicylate is indicated topically for the treatment of glaucomas and is also a valuable drug for treating toxicity of anticholinergic drugs such as atropine. Malathion is an anticholinesterase that is used topically for the treatment of head lice and is never used internally.

307. The answer is D. *(DiPalma, 4/e, pp 368, 371. Gilman, 8/e, pp 216, 316–317.)* The addition of a vasoconstrictor, such as epinephrine or phenylephrine, to certain short-acting, local anesthetics is a common practice in order to prevent the rapid systemic absorption of the local anesthetic, to prolong the local action, and to decrease the potential systemic reactions. Some local anesthetics cause vasodilation, which allows more compound to escape the tissue and enter the blood. Procaine (Novocaine) is an ester-type local anesthetic with a short duration of action due to rather rapid biotransformation in the plasma by cholinesterases. The duration of action of the drug during infiltration anesthesia is greatly increased by the addition of epinephrine, which reduces the vasodilation caused by procaine.

308. The answer is D. *(DiPalma, 4/e, p 176. Gilman, 8/e, p 173.)* Flaccid paralysis of all skeletal muscles can be produced by the intravenous administration of large doses of a neuromuscular blocking agent such as tubocurarine. However, not all skeletal musculature is equally sensitive to the action of these drugs. The muscles that produce fine movements—e.g., the extraocular muscles, fingers, and muscles of the head, face, and neck—are most sensitive to these drugs. Muscles of the trunk, abdomen, and extremities are relaxed next, and the respiratory muscles, i.e., the intercostals and the diaphragm, are the most resistant to the action of tubocurarine.

309. The answer is A. *(AMA Drug Evaluations Annual, 1993, pp 1834–1835.)* Epinephrine is the drug of choice to relieve the symptoms of an acute, systemic, immediate hypersensitivity reaction to an allergen (anaphylactic shock). Subcutaneous administration of a 1:1000 solution of epinephrine rapidly relieves itching and urticaria and may save the life of the patient when laryngeal edema and bronchospasm threaten suffocation and severe hypotension and cardiac arrhythmias become life-endangering. Norepinephrine, isoproterenol, and atropine are ineffective therapies. Angioedema is responsive to antihistamines (e.g., diphenhydramine), but epinephrine is necessary in the event of a severe reaction.

310. The answer is A. *(AMA Drug Evaluations Annual, 1993, pp 576–578. DiPalma, 4/e, pp 139–140, 143, 475–476.)* Phentolamine is a nonselective alpha-adrenergic receptor blocker; i.e., it has affinity for both $alpha_1$- and $alpha_2$-adrenergic receptor sites. It also has a prominent direct relaxant (musculotropic spasmolytic) effect on arterioles, which results in vasodilation and reflex tachycardia. In addition, phentolamine can block the effects of serotonin and will increase hydrochloric acid and pepsin secretion from the stomach. Phentolamine is used for the short-term control of hypertension in patients with pheochromocytoma (i.e., a type of secondary hypertension); owing to the high incidence of tachycardia associated with the compound, it is not used chronically for the treatment of primary hypertension.

Prazosin is a selective $alpha_1$-adrenergic receptor antagonist that, at therapeutic doses, has little activity at $alpha_2$-adrenergic receptors and clinically insignificant direct vasodilating activity. The drug does not cause the other effects attributed to phentolamine. Most importantly, it produces less tachycardia than does phentolamine and, therefore, is useful in the treatment of primary hypertension.

311. The answer is C. *(DiPalma, 4/e, p 177.)* Unlike most other neuromuscular blocking agents, cardioacceleration may be observed with both pancuronium bromide and gallamine triethiodide (Flaxedil). The increased heart rate that may be observed with pancuronium appears to be primarily due to an atropine-like antimuscarinic (vagolytic) action on the heart, although other mechanisms have been proposed including (1) release of catecholamines from postganglionic adrenergic cardiac fibers, (2) blockade of neuronal norepinephrine reuptake, and (3) a mild ganglionic (N_M) stimulant effect. Pancuronium does not cause hypotension, has little ganglionic blocking activity, does not affect the myocardium like digitalis, and does not cross the blood-brain barrier in order to stimulate the vasomotor center.

312. The answer is D. *(DiPalma, 4/e, pp 151–153. Gilman, 8/e, pp 180–181.)* Nicotine is a depolarizing ganglionic blocking agent; that is, it stimulates nicotinic receptors in low doses and predominantly blocks at high dose levels. The effect of nicotine on a particular tissue or organ depends on the relative contribution to function made by each division of the autonomic nervous system. The effects on the cardiovascular system are complex. Stimulation of the cardiac vagal ganglia causes bradycardia. This is countered by sympathetic stimulation to the heart (tachycardia), blood vessels (vasoconstriction), and adrenal medulla (catecholamine release: tachycardia and vasoconstriction). Thus the net effect of nicotine on the heart is tachycardia, not bradycardia. Low doses of nicotine augment respiration by excitation of the chemoreceptors of the carotid body and aortic arch. Higher doses also stimulate the medullary respiratory center and increase respiration through CNS activity. Large amounts of nicotine cause respiratory failure from medullary paralysis and blockade of the skeletal muscles of respiration.

313. The answer is B. *(DiPalma, 4/e, pp 158, 194, 277, 278, 292, 293.)* Many compounds from diverse pharmacologic categories elicit antimuscarinic (anticholinergic) effects. As an example, diphenhydramine (an antihistamine), meperidine (an opioid analgesic), amitriptyline (an antidepressant), and thioridazine (an antipsychotic) all produce clinically significant antimuscarinic effects. In some cases, these become annoying adverse reactions, e.g., dryness of the mouth and tachycardia, as seen with amitriptyline. In other instances this property can be useful; e.g., reduced nasal secretions enhance the utility of diphenhydramine in the therapy of colds and allergies.

Pyridostigmine does not have antimuscarinic activity; rather, it *produces* muscarinic and nicotinic effects. This drug is an indirect-acting cholinomimetic agent that inhibits the activity of acetylcholinesterase and plasma cholinesterase, the enzymes that hydrolyze acetylcholine. Pyridostigmine is used as the drug of choice for oral therapy of myasthenia gravis.

314. The answer is A. *(DiPalma, 4/e, pp 177–179.)* Many of the older neuromuscular blocking agents, such as tubocurarine chloride, metocurine iodide (Metubine Iodide), and gallamine triethiodide (Flaxedil) are very stable in the body and therefore are not biotransformed to a significant extent; these drugs are eliminated unchanged from the body primarily via the kidney. Doxacurium chloride (Nuromax) is a newer neuromuscular blocking agent that is not biotransformed; its routes of elimination are through the bile and urine. Most of the other neuromuscular blocking drugs are biotransformed by either deacetylation or by hydrolysis of ester groups. Pancuronium, pipecuronium, and vecuronium are partially deacetylated to the active products 3-hydroxy pancuronium, 3-desacetyl pipecuronium, and 3-desacetyl vecuronium, respectively. Succinylcholine is hydrolyzed by cholinesterases to form succinylmonocholine, an active skeletal muscle relaxant. Atracurium and mivacurium chloride (Mivacron) are metabolized by ester hydrolysis to inactive products.

315. The answer is D. *(DiPalma, 4/e, pp 114–119, 121–122. Gilman, 8/e, pp 201–202.)* Isoproterenol is a nonselective beta-adrenergic receptor agonist. Cardiac stimulation (via $beta_1$-receptors), relaxed bronchial smooth muscle, and vasodilation (via $beta_2$-receptors) are typical effects observed following the administration of the drug. Based on these effects, isoproterenol is used as a cardiac stimulant in heart block and shock (by injection) and as a bronchodilator in respiratory disorders (by inhalation). The drug is short-acting since it is metabolized primarily and efficiently by catechol-*O*-methyltransferase (COMT). It is a relatively poor substrate for MAO, however.

316. The answer is E. *(DiPalma, 4/e, p 136. Gilman, 8/e, pp 238–239.)* Propranolol is a competitive antagonist of both $beta_1$- and $beta_2$-adrenergic receptors. Since the sympathetic division of the autonomic nervous system may be a vital component in support of cardiac performance in many patients with congestive heart failure, $beta_1$-adrenergic blockade may precipitate more severe depression of cardiac function. The $beta_2$-adrenoceptors in the bronchioles of patients with bronchospastic disease (e.g., bronchial asthma, chronic bronchitis, emphysema) are important in mediating bronchodilation; thus, blockade of these receptors may cause a severe increase in airway resistance, thereby decreasing pulmonary function in such patients, which may be life-threatening. Propranolol should also be used with caution in diabetic patients who are prone to hypoglycemia since beta-adrenergic blockers may mask the warning signs of acute hypoglycemia (e.g., tachycardia). Some patients who use propranolol and other beta-adrenergic blockers complain of cold extremities. Since these drugs may mildly elevate peripheral resistance, they should be used with caution in patients with vasospastic diseases such as Raynaud's phenomenon and acrocyanosis. There is no contraindication or warning concerning the use of propranolol in angina pectoris; rather, propranolol and other beta-adrenergic blocking agents are indicated for the treatment of this disease. There have been reports, however, of exacerbation of angina following abrupt discontinuation of these drugs.

317. The answer is B. *(DiPalma, 4/e, pp 102–103. Gilman, 8/e, pp 89–90.)* The radial muscle of the iris contains predominantly alpha-adrenergic receptors; when exposed to such alpha-receptor agonists as phenylephrine, the muscle contracts, resulting in mydriasis. Miosis occurs when the ciliary muscle, which contains beta-receptors, relaxes. Bronchial muscle, the atrioventricular node, and the sinoatrial node are among other sites that contain beta-receptors and respond to beta-adrenergic agonists.

318. The answer is C. *(DiPalma, 4/e, pp 131, 143–145, 318. Gilman, 8/e, pp 475, 794–796.)* Selegiline (also known as *deprenyl*) is a selective monoamine oxidase (MAO) inhibitor that is used to treat Parkinson's disease. At recommended doses, the drug inhibits MAO type B (found mainly in the brain), with little effect on MAO type A (found predominantly in the intestine and liver). Inhibition of MAO will tend to raise the pool of catecholamine neurotransmitters (norepinephrine, dopamine) available for release by sympathetic neurons.

Guanadrel and guanethidine are adrenergic neuronal blocking drugs that deplete stores of neurotransmitters in sympathetic neurons by competing with catecholamine for binding sites within the storage vesicles. When the sympathetic neurons are depolarized, less neurotransmitter is available to be released. Both of these compounds are used to treat essential hypertension.

Reserpine causes depletion of norepinephrine and dopamine by binding to the membrane of the storage vesicles and irreversibly inhibiting the magnesium-dependent ATP transport process that is responsible for catecholamine uptake into the neuronal vesicles. Like guanethidine and guanadrel, reserpine is indicated for the treatment of essential hypertension.

Metyrosine is a competitive antagonist of tyrosine hydroxylase, the enzyme that converts tyrosine to dihydroxyphenylalanine (DOPA), and the rate-limiting step in the formation of norepinephrine and epinephrine. Metyrosine is used to treat patients with pheochromocytoma, a tumor of the adrenal medulla that produces excessive quantities of these catecholamines and results in hypertension. This compound is not recommended for use in essential hypertension or in hypertension secondary to diseases other than functional adrenal tumors.

319. The answer is E. *(DiPalma, 4/e, p 125. Gilman, 8/e, pp 200–201.)* Dopamine is a mixed-acting sympathomimetic drug that complexes with and activates alpha- and beta$_1$-adrenergic receptors and induces norepinephrine release from sympathetic neurons. Dopamine is unique in that is has little agonistic activity on beta$_2$-adrenergic receptors, but it is a potent stimulant of dopaminergic receptor sites. At low concentrations, activation of D_1-dopaminergic receptors in the renal vasculature mediates vasodilation and increased blood flow in this area, resulting in an enhancement of renal function. At somewhat higher concentrations, myocardial beta$_1$-adrenergic receptors are stimulated, resulting in an increased force of contraction; high concentrations of the drug activate vascular alpha-adrenoceptors, which mediate vasoconstriction. Thus dopamine is used for patients with oliguria, with low peripheral resistance, and with some types of shock, e.g., cardiogenic and septic shock. Although dopamine receptors are present in the central nervous system (CNS), the drug does not cross the blood-brain barrier to any significant extent; therefore, CNS adverse reactions are uncommonly observed in most patients. Since dopamine is a catecholamine, it is rapidly inactivated by hepatic monoamine oxidase and catechol-*O*-methyltransferase and, therefore, must be administered by intravenous infusion.

320. The answer is D. *(DiPalma, 4/e, pp 164–166. Gilman, 8/e, pp 154–157.)* Acetylcholine will stimulate both muscarinic and nicotinic receptors. Ganglionic stimulation is an effect of nicotinic-neural (N_N) receptors and skeletal muscle contraction is mediated through nicotinic-muscular (N_M) receptors. All the other effects listed in the question occur following muscarinic receptor activation and will be blocked by atropine and scopolamine, both of which are muscarinic receptor antagonists. Skeletal muscle contraction will not be affected by these drugs; rather, a neuromuscular blocker (e.g., tubocurarine) is required to antagonize this effect of acetylcholine.

321. The answer is D. *(DiPalma, 4/e, pp 123–124. Gilman, 8/e, pp 205, 632–633.)* Beta-adrenergic receptors are regulatory subunits of adenylate cyclase, the intracellular enzyme that converts adenosine triphosphate (ATP) to cyclic AMP. Selective beta$_2$-adrenergic receptor stimulants (e.g., albuterol, isoetharine, metaproterenol, terbutaline) as well as the nonselective beta-receptor agonists (epinephrine and isoproterenol) all enhance the activity of this enzyme. Like all sympathomimetics, terbutaline and isoetharine elicit CNS side effects, muscle tremors, and, although less than the nonselective beta-receptor agonists, tachycardia. Although the metabolism of each compound is different, extensive first-pass biotransformation of both drugs will occur following oral administration. Isoetharine is a catecholamine, biotransformed by catechol-*O*-methyltransferase (COMT) and is effective only by inhalation. Terbutaline is not biotransformed by COMT, but significant biotransformation via hepatic microsomal enzymes occurs (the oral bioavailability is only about 15 percent). Despite this, oral doses are large enough to compensate and the drug is effective when given orally.

322. The answer is C. *(DiPalma, 4/e, p 138. Gilman, 8/e, pp 234, 239–240.)* In addition to its usefulness in the treatment of hypertension, angina pectoris, supraventricular and ventricular arrhythmias, and in the prophylaxis of migraine headaches, propranolol is indicated for use in hypertrophic subaortic stenosis and pheochromocytoma and to reduce cardiovascular mortality following a myocardial infarction. Propranolol is the beta-adrenergic blocker with the greatest *membrane stabilizing activity* (also known as *local anesthetic activity*). Propranolol applied topically to membranes, such as the cornea, would anesthetize the area; in the case of the eye, this would be detrimental to the patient. Therefore, this drug is not used for the treatment of glaucoma. Other beta-adrenergic blockers that do not have membrane stabilizing activity—including timolol (Timoptic), betaxolol (Betoptic), and levobunolol (Betagen)—are useful for this purpose. All of these are administered as drops to the eye.

323. The answer is A. *(DiPalma, 4/e, pp 127, 268–269. Gilman, 8/e, pp 210–213, 217–218.)* Amphetamine and its derivative methamphetamine are sympathomimetic compounds that promote the release of various biogenic amines (e.g., dopamine, norepinephrine, serotonin) from storage vesicles in neurons and are agonists at alpha- and beta-adrenergic receptor sites. Oral administration of amphetamine *raises* both systolic and diastolic blood pressure and may cause heart rate to slow reflexly. The drug is a potent CNS stimulant and evokes excitation, increased alertness, elevation of mood, and insomnia. Anorexia (a loss of appetite) is a common manifestation of amphetamine use and the drug is widely used in the treatment of obesity, although such use is questionable owing to the high potential for abuse of the compound. Amphetamine is approved for use in narcolepsy, a disease characterized by sudden attacks of sleep, and in attention-deficit hyperactivity disorder, a syndrome in children characterized by impulsive behavior, short attention span, and excessive motor activity.

324. The answer is D. *(DiPalma, 4/e, pp 126–127. Gilman, 8/e, pp 213–214.)* Ephedrine directly stimulates both alpha- and beta-adrenergic receptors and causes release of norepinephrine from adrenergic neurons. Qualitatively its pharmacologic effects resemble those of epinephrine; the drug can increase blood pressure by both vasoconstriction and cardiac stimulation and it will relax bronchiolar smooth muscle. Ephedrine is less potent than epinephrine and the effects observed are usually slower in onset and of longer duration than those of epinephrine. Also in contrast to epinephrine, ephedrine is used orally in many cough and cold preparations for its decongestant activity.

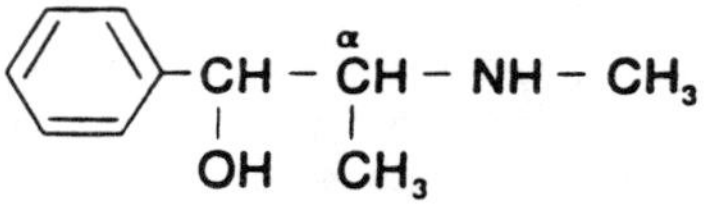

Ephedrine is quite lipid-soluble compared with epinephrine and will pass through the blood-brain barrier and may cause stimulation of the CNS. Since epinephrine lacks a catechol moiety, it is not biotransformed by COMT and the methyl substitution on the alpha carbon allows the drug to resist oxidation by MAO.

325. The answer is E. *(DiPalma, 4/e, pp 170–172.)* Mecamylamine is a competitive antagonist of acetylcholine at ganglionic cholinergic receptors (N_N) and will reduce the activity of both the parasympathetic and the sympathetic divisions of the autonomic nervous system. Since the sympathetic nervous system controls vascular reactivity, mecamylamine will block sympathetic tone to the arterioles, resulting in vasodilation and decreased blood pressure; because of this effect, the drug is used (although rarely today) for the treatment of chronic hypertension. Parasympathetic tone predominates at most other effector structures and, therefore, this drug will affect the heart (tachycardia), eye (mydriasis and cycloplegia), gastrointestinal tract (constipation), urinary bladder (retention of urine), salivary glands (xerostomia), and sweat glands (anhidrosis); these are all adverse manifestations of the compound. Since the nerve pathway to skeletal muscle involves only a single cholinergic motor nerve and no ganglia, and since mecamylamine does not compete with acetylcholine for binding to N_M receptors at the myoneural junction, mecamylamine will have no effect on skeletal muscle tone.

326. The answer is B. *(AMA Drug Evaluations Annual, 1993, pp 672–673. DiPalma, 4/e, pp 122–123.)* At low therapeutic doses, this catecholamine is a selective agonist of myocardial ($beta_1$-adrenergic) receptors; in higher doses, it will lose selectivity and stimulate $beta_2$- and alpha-adrenergic receptor sites. Although it is a structural derivative of dopamine, dobutamine has no activity on peripheral dopaminergic receptors.

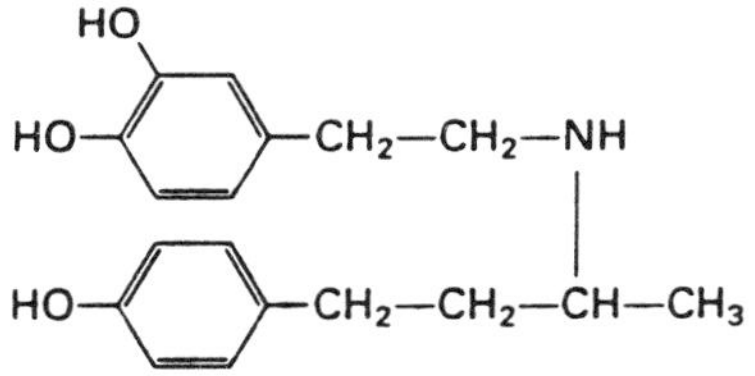

Dobutamine

The drug is not effective orally since it is rapidly biotransformed (plasma $t_{1/2}$ is approximately 2 min) by catechol-*O*-methyltransferase (COMT) and, therefore, must be given by intravenous infusion. It is used to improve myocardial function in patients with severe cardiac failure that has not responded to other treatment modalities. Cardiac adverse effects (e.g., tachycardia and anginal pain) may be observed and represent extensions of the pharmacologic activity of the drug.

327. The answer is C. *(Gilman, 8/e, pp 88–90.)* Cholinergic impulses arising from the parasympathetic division of the autonomic nervous system affect many tissues and organs throughout the body. Physiologically, this system is concerned primarily with the functions of energy conservation and maintenance of organ function during periods of reduced activity. Slowed heart rate, reduced blood pressure, increased gastrointestinal motility, emptying of the urinary bladder, and stimulation of secretions from the pancreas, salivary glands, lacrimal glands, and bronchial and nasopharyngeal glands are all effects observed due to activation of this nervous system. However, skeletal muscle contraction is mediated through activation of the somatic nervous system, not the autonomic nervous system.

328. The answer is E. *(Gilman, 8/e, pp 116–118.)* Although acetylcholine and norepinephrine are still considered the major neurotransmitters in the parasympathetic and sympathetic divisions of the autonomic nervous system, respectively, other compounds that exist within autonomic nerve terminals have been found to be released simultaneously during nerve stimulation and are now viewed as cotransmitters or neuromodulators. For example, VIP is localized in a number of parasympathetic neurons, e.g., those that innervate sweat glands and salivary glands, and it appears to function as a cotransmitter with acetylcholine in these structures. ATP and acetylcholine both exist in cholinergic vesicles, and ATP is found within the granules of adrenergic fibers and in the adrenal medulla; this compound is believed to be a neurotransmitter in the gastrointestinal and genitourinary tracts. NPY appears associated with catecholamine-containing neurons and may contribute to vasoconstriction produced by stimulation of the sympathetic nervous system. Although less is known about the function of substance P, this small peptide is found within cholinergic nerves, especially at ganglionic sites, and may function as a neuromodulator. Serotonin (5-hydroxytryptamine) is a neurotransmitter in the CNS; although it may play a role in regulating gastrointestinal motility via peripheral serotonergic neurons, it has not been designated as a cotransmitter or neuromodulator in the autonomic nervous system.

329–331. The answers are 329-I, 330-F, 331-B. *(DiPalma, 4/e, pp 130–132, 138, 143, 173–175, 475. Gilman, 8/e, pp 150–153, 169–174, 226–227, 235.)* Timolol is a beta-adrenergic receptor antagonist. It does not show selectivity for $beta_1$- or $beta_2$-adrenoceptors and, therefore, decreases heart rate by blocking the action of endogenous catecholamines. Timolol, used to lower intraocular pressure in patients with chronic open-angle glaucoma, presumably by decreasing the production of aqueous humor, is more effective than many other types of drugs in the treatment of glaucoma.

Atracurium is a nondepolarizing neuromuscular blocking agent. Similar to tubocurarine, atracurium is a competitive antagonist of acetylcholine at N_M receptors at the myoneural junction of skeletal muscle. At therapeutic doses, these drugs can induce complete paralysis of skeletal muscles, unlike the weaker, centrally acting skeletal muscle relaxants (e.g., diazepam, baclofen, and cyclobenzaprine), which reduce muscular spasms but do not completely block skeletal muscle contractions. The primary therapeutic use of atracurium and other curariform drugs is as an adjunct in surgical anesthesia to relax the skeletal musculature so that surgical manipulations are facilitated.

Doxazosin is a reversible blocker of postsynaptic $alpha_1$-adrenergic receptors, unlike phenoxybenzamine or phentolamine, which are nonselective and react at both presynaptic ($alpha_2$) and postsynaptic ($alpha_1$) receptors. Doxazosin, like its congeners prazosin and terazosin, is used to treat primary hypertension (whereas nonselective alpha-adrenergic antagonists are not) because the drug does not significantly block the negative feedback at presynaptic nerve terminals. When this negative feedback mechanism is blocked by nonselective antagonists, the resulting increase in secretion of the catecholamine neurotransmitter norepinephrine causes a significant increase in heart rate, which is an unacceptable adverse effect in the hypertensive patient.

332–334. The answers are 332-D, 333-C, 334-A. *(Gilman, 8/e, pp 257–262.)* Dopamine is formed from tyrosine by hydroxylation with tyrosine hydroxylase and the removal of a CO_2 group by aromatic amino acid decarboxylase. The catecholamine is found in high concentrations in parts of the brain: the caudate nucleus, the median eminence, the tuberculum olfactorium, and the nucleus accumbens. Dopamine appears to act as an inhibitory neurotransmitter.

Norepinephrine is synthesized from dopamine by dopamine-β-oxidase, which hydroxylates the β-carbon. This enzyme is localized in the amine storage granules. Norepinephrine is found in adrenergic fibers, the adrenal medulla, and in neurons in the locus ceruleus and lateral ventral tegmental fields of the central nervous system.

Epinephrine is synthesized from norepinephrine in the adrenal medulla. Norepinephrine is methylated by phenylethanolamine-*N*-methyltransferase. Neurons containing this enzyme are also found in the central nervous system.

335–337. The answers are 335-C, 336-E, 337-I. *(DiPalma, 4/e, pp 130–133, 143–144, 299–300. Gilman, 8/e, pp 103, 229, 237, 414–415, 795.)* Reserpine is an adrenergic neuronal blocking agent that causes depletion of central and peripheral stores of norepinephrine and dopamine. Reserpine acts by irreversibly inhibiting the magnesium-dependent ATP transport process that functions as a carrier for biogenic amines from the cytoplasm of the neuron into the storage vesicle. Depletion of stored norepinephrine results in decreased sympathetic tone; therefore, reserpine causes vasodilation, bradycardia, and hypotension.

Esmolol hydrochloride (Brevibloc) is a competitive beta-adrenergic receptor antagonist; it is selective for $beta_1$-adrenoceptors. In contrast to pindolol, esmolol has little intrinsic sympathomimetic activity, and it differs from propranolol in that it lacks membrane stabilizing activity. Of all the beta-adrenergic blocking drugs, this compound has the shortest duration of action; since it is an ester, it is hydrolyzed rapidly by plasma esterases and must be used by the intravenous route. Esmolol is approved only for the treatment of supraventricular arrhythmias.

Tranylcypromine sulfate (Parnate) is an antidepressant drug and an inhibitor of monoamine oxidase (MAO). Its antidepressant effect is probably due to the accumulation of norepinephrine in the brain as a consequence of inhibition of the enzyme. The other monoamine oxidase inhibitor currently used as an antidepressant is phenelzine sulfate (Nardil).

338–340. The answers are 338-A, 339-D, 340-E. *(DiPalma, 4/e, pp 117, 148, 186.)* Acetylcholine, which serves as the neurotransmitter at some synapses within the central nervous system, at autonomic ganglia, and at many peripheral neuroeffector sites, is an ester formed within the cholinergic neuron by the acetylation of choline. The acetylation reaction is catalyzed by the enzyme choline acetyltransferase (choline acetylase). After its release, acetylcholine is usually rapidly hydrolyzed by the enzyme acetylcholinesterase.

Dopamine (C) is the neurotransmitter at selected synapses within the central nervous system and probably within some autonomic ganglia. It is formed within the neuron by the ring hydroxylation of phenylalanine and the subsequent decarboxylation of the resultant dihydroxyphenylalanine. Routes of metabolism of neuronally released dopamine include oxidation by monoamine oxidase and aldehyde dehydrogenase to 3,4-dihydroxyphenylacetic acid and methylation by catechol-*O*-methyltransferase to 3-methoxydopamine.

Norepinephrine (B) is the principal neurotransmitter at peripheral autonomic adrenergic neuroeffector junctions, is synthesized within the adrenergic neuron by the β-hydroxylation of dopamine, and—in contrast to epinephrine—lacks the methyl substituent in the amino group. Much of the neuronally released norepinephrine reenters the adrenergic neuron; reentry into the cell is accomplished by a specific, active transport system.

Histamine is a naturally occurring substance involved in anaphylaxis and allergic reactions. It is formed by the decarboxylation of histidine and is catabolized by two routes: one involving oxidative deamination with subsequent conjugation with ribose, and the other involving ring methylation with subsequent side-chain oxidation.

Epinephrine is a catecholamine released by the adrenal medulla. It is formed by *N*-methylation of norepinephrine, a reaction catalyzed by the enzyme phenylethanolamine-*N*-methyltransferase. In large part, circulating epinephrine is methylated by catechol-*O*-methyltransferase, and the resultant metanephrine undergoes oxidative deamination by monoamine oxidase to yield 3-methoxy-4-hydroxymandelic acid.

341–343. The answers are 341-A, 342-C, 343-D. *(DiPalma, 4/e, pp 107, 186, 200. Gilman, 8/e, pp 102, 576, 592–593.)* Epinephrine is made from tyrosine in a series of steps through dopa, dopamine, norepinephrine, and finally epinephrine. The conversion of tyrosine to dopa by tyrosine hydroxylase is the rate-limiting step in this pathway. Epinephrine constitutes about 80 percent of the catecholamines in the adrenal medulla. The enzyme that synthesizes epinephrine from norepinephrine is also found in certain areas of the central nervous system.

Histamine, formed by the decarboxylation of histidine, is stored in mast cells and basophils; some other tissues can synthesize histamine but do not store it. Histamine is released from sensitized mast cells during allergic reactions.

Serotonin (5-hydroxytryptamine) is synthesized from tryptophan in two steps. Tryptophan is hydroxylated by tryptophan hydroxylase, and 5-hydroxytryptophan is decarboxylated to give serotonin. Most serotonin in the body is found in the enterochromaffin cells of the intestinal tract and the pineal gland. Platelets take up and store serotonin but do not synthesize it.

344–346. The answers are 344-E, 345-C, 346-B. *(DiPalma, 4/e, pp 128, 144–145, 168–169. Gilman, 8/e, pp 161–163, 217–218, 794–795.)* Guanethidine inhibits the activity of peripheral sympathetic nerves by impairing neurotransmitter (norepinephrine) release. Chronic administration causes depletion of norepinephrine from intraneuronal storage granules by displacement. Reduced activity of the sympathetic division of the autonomic nervous system leads to bradycardia, vasodilation, and reduced systemic blood pressure.

Propantheline is a semisynthetic antimuscarinic agent, similar to atropine and scopolamine. Its major use is in the treatment of peptic ulcer and gastrointestinal hypermotility. Although less potent than atropine for this purpose, it will produce adverse effects commonly associated with the antimuscarinic group, e.g., xerostomia, tachycardia, and dilated pupils.

Methylphenidate is structurally and pharmacologically related to amphetamine. It is used in both children and adults who are characterized as having attention-deficit disorder (ADD). It has been found to be effective in improving behavior, concentration, and learning ability in 70 to 80 percent of children with ADD. Like amphetamine, it is a CNS stimulant and has significant potential for abuse.

347–349. The answers are 347-C, 348-A, 349-D. *(DiPalma, 4/e, pp 104–106, 150–151.)* Acetylcholine is synthesized from acetyl-CoA and choline. Choline is taken up into the neurons by an active transport system. Hemicholinium blocks this uptake, depleting cellular choline, so that synthesis of acetylcholine no longer occurs.

Botulinus toxin comes from *Clostridium botulinum*, an organism that causes food poisoning. Botulinus toxin prevents the release of acetylcholine from nerve endings by mechanisms that are not clear. Death occurs from respiratory failure caused by the inability of diaphragm muscles to contract.

Muscarine, an alkaloid from certain species of mushrooms, is a muscarinic receptor agonist. The compound has toxicologic importance; muscarine poisoning will produce all the effects associated with an overdose of acetylcholine, e.g., bronchoconstriction, bradycardia, hypotension, excessive salivary and respiratory secretion, and sweating. Poisoning by muscarine is treated with atropine.

Local Control Substances

- Ibuprofen
- Ketoprofen
- Naproxen
- Oxaprozin

Acetic acids

- Indomethacin
- Sulindac
- Tolmetin
- Diclofenac

Oxicams

- Piroxicam

Pyrazolone

- Phenylbutazone

Fenamates

- Meclofenamate
- Mefenamic acid

DIRECTIONS: Each question below contains five suggested responses. Select the **one best** response to each question.

350. Sumatriptan succinate (Imitrex) is effective for the treatment of acute migraine headaches by acting as

(A) an antagonist at $beta_1$- and $beta_2$-adrenergic receptors
(B) a selective antagonist at H_1 receptors
(C) an inhibitor of prostacyclin synthase
(D) an agonist at nicotinic receptors
(E) a selective agonist at $5\text{-}HT_{1D}$ receptors

351. Presently, three subtypes of histamine receptors are proposed: H_1 and H_2 receptors are found in peripheral tissues and the CNS, and H_3 receptors are found in the CNS. The second messenger pathway that mediates H_1 receptor stimulation is

(A) increased formation of inositol trisphosphate
(B) elevation of intracellular cyclic AMP
(C) activation of tyrosine kinases
(D) inhibition of adenylate cyclase activity
(E) activation of sodium ion flow into the cell

352. The pharmacologic effects of acetylsalicylic acid include

(A) a reduction in elevated body temperature
(B) promotion of platelet aggregation
(C) alleviation of pain by stimulation of prostaglandin synthesis
(D) efficacy equal to that of acetaminophen as an anti-inflammatory agent
(E) less gastric irritation than other salicylates

353. Which of the following is used in the treatment of acute migraine headaches because of its vasoconstrictor properties?

(A) Ergotamine (Ergostat)
(B) Propranolol (Inderal)
(C) Methysergide (Sansert)
(D) Pseudoephedrine (Sudafed)
(E) Aspirin

354. Cyproheptadine (Periactin) is an antagonist at

(A) dopamine (D_1) receptors
(B) nicotine (N_N) receptors
(C) benzodiazepine (BZ) receptors
(D) histamine (H_2) receptors
(E) serotonin (5-HT) receptors

DIRECTIONS: Each numbered question or incomplete statement is NEGATIVELY phrased. Select the **one best** lettered response.

355. Which of the following H_1 receptor antagonists (antihistamines) causes the LEAST sedation at therapeutic doses?

(A) Hydroxyzine (Atarax)
(B) Diphenhydramine (Benadryl)
(C) Terfenadine (Seldane)
(D) Promethazine (Phenergan)
(E) Tripelennamine (PBZ)

356. Following the administration of aspirin and the inhibition of the activity of the enzyme prostaglandin endoperoxide synthase, the production of all the following products of the arachidonic acid cascade will be reduced EXCEPT

(A) thromboxane A_2
(B) prostaglandin E_2
(C) prostacyclin
(D) leukotriene C_4
(E) prostaglandin $F_{2\alpha}$

357. All the following are therapeutic uses of natural prostaglandins or synthetic prostaglandin derivatives EXCEPT

(A) abortion
(B) cervical ripening in pregnant women
(C) temporary maintenance of the patency of the ductus arteriosus in preterm neonates
(D) prevention of gastric ulceration caused by nonsteroidal anti-inflammatory drugs
(E) treatment of chronic obstructive pulmonary diseases like bronchial asthma

358. All the following drugs are useful for the treatment of inflammatory conditions, e.g., rheumatoid arthritis, EXCEPT

(A) indomethacin (Indocin)
(B) acetaminophen (Tylenol)
(C) tolmetin sodium (Tolectin)
(D) naproxen (Naprosyn)
(E) piroxicam (Feldene)

359. All the following are effects of serotonin (5-hydroxytryptamine, 5-HT) EXCEPT

(A) increased heart rate and force of contraction
(B) vasoconstriction of arterioles of the pulmonary and renal beds
(C) stimulation of pain and itching responses
(D) contraction of bronchial smooth muscle
(E) relaxation of gastrointestinal smooth muscle

Local Control Substances

Answers

350. The answer is E. *(DiPalma, 4/e, pp 201–202. Katzung, 6/e, p 265.)* Sumatriptan is closely related to serotonin (5-hydroxytryptamine, 5-HT) in structure and it is believed that the drug is effective in the treatment of acute migraine headaches by virtue of its selective agonistic activity at 5-HT_{1D} receptors. These receptors, present on cerebral and meningeal arteries, mediate vasoconstriction induced by 5-HT. In addition, 5-HT_{1D} receptors are found on presynaptic nerve terminals and function to inhibit the release of neuropeptides and other neurotransmitters. It has been suggested that the pain of migraine headaches is caused by vasodilation of intracranial blood vessels and stimulation of trigeminovascular axons, which cause pain and release vasoactive neuropeptides to produce neurogenic inflammation and edema. Sumatriptan acts to reduce vasodilation and the release of neurotransmitters and, therefore, reduces the pain associated with migraine headaches. Other antimigraine drugs, e.g., ergotamine and dihydroergotamine, also exhibit high affinities for the 5-HT_{1D} receptor site.

351. The answer is A. *(DiPalma, 4/e, pp 188–189. Katzung, 6/e, pp 252–253.)* H_1 receptors appear to be linked to phospholipase C; activation of these receptors results in an increase in the intracellular formation of inositol-1,4,5-trisphosphate (IP_3) and 1,2-diacylglycerol. IP_3 binds to a receptor located on the endoplasmic reticulum, initiating the release of calcium into the cytosol, where it activates calcium-dependent protein kinases. Diacylglycerol activates protein kinase C. Additionally, stimulation of H_1 receptors may activate phospholipase A_2 and trigger the arachidonic acid cascade, leading to prostaglandin production.

H_2 receptors are associated with adenylate cyclase and stimulation of these receptors increases the cytosolic concentration of cyclic AMP and activation of cyclic AMP–dependent protein kinase. Although inhibition of adenylate cyclase has been suggested as the intracellular signaling mechanism associated with H_3 receptors, this has not been completely substantiated.

352. The answer is A. *(DiPalma, 4/e, pp 345–353. Katzung, 6/e, pp 538–542.)* Aspirin (acetylsalicyclic acid) is the most extensively used analgesic, antipyretic, and anti-inflammatory agent of the group of compounds known as *nonsteroidal anti-inflammatory drugs (NSAIDs)*, or *nonopioid anal-*

gesics. Most of its therapeutic and adverse effects appear to be related to the inhibition of prostaglandin synthesis. NSAIDs inhibit the activity of the enzyme cyclooxygenase, which mediates the conversion of arachidonic acid to prostaglandins that are involved in pain, fever, and inflammation. Aspirin may produce irritation and ulceration of the gastrointestinal tract, an adverse effect that is about equal to other salicylates. It also inhibits platelet aggregation. Acetaminophen, like aspirin, has analgesic and antipyretic properties but does not have clinically significant anti-inflammatory activity and is not irritating to the gastrointestinal tract.

353. The answer is A. *(DiPalma, 4/e, pp 202–203. Gilman, 8/e, pp 945–947.)* Ergotamine has several pharmacologic properties, including blockade of alpha-adrenergic receptors; however, its mechanism of action in treating migraine headaches is primarily related to its agonistic interaction with 5-HT_{1D} receptors, resulting in vasoconstriction. Ergotamine is the drug of choice for combating an incipient attack of migraine headache. Although chronic treatment with this nonsedative, nonanalgesic drug does not decrease the frequency of or prevent migraine attacks, the administration of oral doses is recommended at the beginning of an attack, especially during the prodromal stage. Its use in this setting is recommended despite its low oral bioavailability, which is due to high first-pass hepatic biotransformation, and the fact that its effects are much slower with oral than with parenteral administration. Ergotamine is often combined with caffeine, which enhances the oral absorption of ergotamine and also has vasoconstricting activity in the central nervous system. Oral ergotamine provides relief in a few minutes and is generally the preferred route for the treatment of mild attacks. Administration of this ergot alkaloid at the peak of a migraine episode requires that doses larger than those administered during the prodromal stage be used and is often associated with a delayed onset of action and a higher incidence of adverse effects, such as nausea, vomiting, pruritus, and disturbances in heart rate.

Propranolol (a beta-adrenergic receptor blocker) and methysergide (a 5-HT receptor antagonist) are used prophylactically to treat migraine headaches, but are not very effective for reducing the pain of migraine headache during an acute attack; furthermore, these drugs do not appear to reduce the pain of migraine headache by vasoconstriction. Nonopioid analgesics, e.g., aspirin, may provide nonspecific symptomatic relief for mild migraine headaches, but are generally not very useful for this type of headache. Vasoconstrictors, e.g., pseudoephedrine, are used as nasal decongestants and have no effect on migraine headaches.

354. The answer is E. *(DiPalma, 4/e, p 203. Katzung, 6/e, pp 257, 265.)* Cyproheptadine is a potent antagonist at serotonin (5-HT) and histamine (H_1)

receptors; in addition, high doses will block muscarinic receptor sites. The drug has no activity at H_2, adrenergic, dopaminergic, nicotinic, or benzodiazepine receptors. Clinically, cyproheptadine is used as an antihistamine for allergic conditions, e.g., allergic rhinitis, urticaria, and pruritus. Due to its ability to inhibit the activity of 5-HT receptors, the drug is also useful in treating hypermotility of the gastrointestinal tract associated with carcinoid tumors and in the prophylaxis of severe headaches in children.

355. The answer is C. *(DiPalma, 4/e, pp 193–194. Katzung, 6/e, p 257.)* As a group, H_1-receptor antagonists elicit depressive effects on the central nervous system at therapeutic doses; thus, most of these compounds will cause varying degrees of diminished alertness, slowed reaction time, muscle weakness, mild sedation, and even somnolence. Some of the drugs are more likely to produce these central nervous system manifestations than others, and patients seem to vary in susceptibility and responsiveness. The aminoalkyl ethers are especially liable to produce sedation; for example, diphenhydramine can produce drowsiness in 20 to 50 percent of patients.

In some circumstances, physicians may take advantage of this sedative effect by using one of these drugs as a sedative prior to or after surgery or may prescribe an H_1-receptor antagonist for patients who are having problems sleeping. For example, hydroxyzine and promethazine are indicated for preoperative and postoperative sedation, and diphenhydramine is contained in most over-the-counter (OTC) preparations that aid in sleeping. Tripelennamine, used in patients with allergic rhinitis and other allergies, may cause significant drowsiness in some patients.

Some of the newer antihistamines, e.g., terfenadine, astemizole (Hismanal), and loratadine (Claritin), elicit reduced or minimal sedative effects. For the most part, these drugs do not cross the blood-brain barrier very well at effective therapeutic doses and, therefore, produce a low incidence of central nervous system effects.

356. The answer is D. *(DiPalma, 4/e, pp 205–210. Gilman, 8/e, pp 601–605.)* As is shown in the figure opposite, arachidonic acid is metabolized through a variety of pathways. Three major mammalian lipoxygenases—i.e., 5-, 12-, and 15-lipoxygenase—catalyze the incorporation of a molecule of oxygen into the 5, 12, or 15 positions of arachidonic acid with the formation of the corresponding 5-, 12-, and 15-hydroperoxyeicosatetraenoic acids (HPETEs). The 5-lipoxygenase pathway is especially important since it generates a variety of leukotrienes that are involved in allergic reactions and certain diseases, e.g., bronchial asthma. Activation of the prostaglandin endoperoxide synthase pathway results in the formation of a number of prostaglandins, prostacyclin, and thromboxane A_2. By inhibiting the cyclooxygenase component of prostaglandin endoperoxide synthase, aspirin and other nonsteroidal anti-inflammatory drugs only inhibit this pathway; therefore, the formation of leukotrienes will not be decreased by the administration of aspirin. The figure below is an overall schematic for the biosynthesis of prostaglandins and related eicosanoids. PG = prostaglandins; TX = thromboxane; HPETE = hydroperoxyeicosatetraenoic acid; HETE = hydroxyeicosatetraenoic acid; and LT = leukotriene.

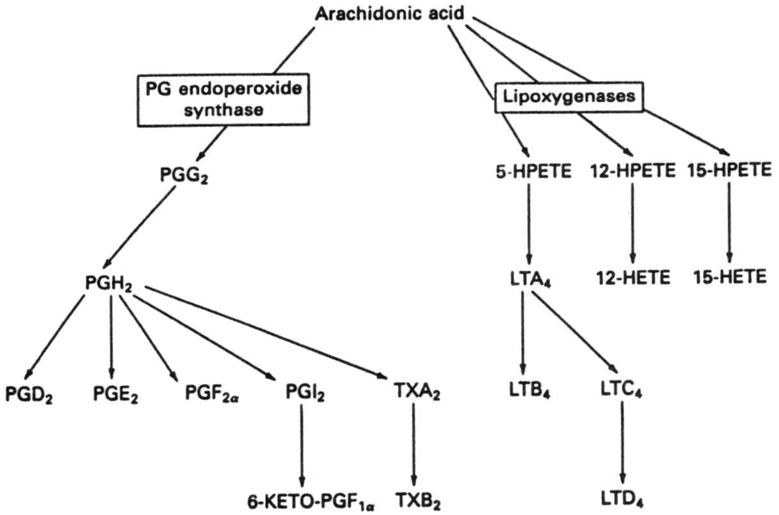

357. The answer is E. *(DiPalma, 4/e, pp 214–215.)* Since they stimulate uterine contraction, both dinoprostone (prostaglandin E_2) and carboprost (15-methyl-prostaglandin $F_{2\alpha}$) are available for use as abortifacients. Typically, dinoprostone (administered by vaginal suppository) and 15-methyl-$PGF_{2\alpha}$ (given by intramuscular injection) are used for therapeutic abortions between the 12th and 20th weeks of gestation. In addition, dinoprostone can be used up to the 28th gestational week when intrauterine fetal death has occurred. Dinoprostone is also indicated for cervical ripening (softening, effacement, and dilation) in pregnant women at or near term who present with a medical or obstetric need to have labor induced; for this purpose, the drug (as a gel) is introduced directly into the cervical canal.

Alprostadil (prostaglandin E_1, PGE_1) is used therapeutically in preterm infants to temporarily maintain the patency of the ductus arteriosus until corrective surgery can be performed. The drug is administered by continuous intravenous infusion or by catheter through the umbilical artery and should only be used in pediatric intensive care facilities. Misoprostol is a synthetic analogue of PGE_1 (15-deoxy-16-hydroxy-16-methyl-PGE_1 methyl ester). It is indicated for the prevention of gastric ulcers in patients taking nonsteroidal anti-inflammatory drugs (e.g., aspirin, indomethacin) and is administered orally.

Some prostaglandins, especially PGE_1, PGE_2, and PGI_2 (prostacyclin), are potent bronchodilators and many prostaglandin analogues have been tested for use in chronic obstructive pulmonary disease. Unfortunately prostaglandins are irritating to the airways and cause coughing when inhaled, which has precluded their use as antiasthmatic drugs. A number of leukotriene antagonists, however, are being examined clinically for use in the treatment of diseases such as bronchial asthma.

358. The answer is B. *(DiPalma, 4/e, pp 347, 354–361. Gilman, 8/e, pp 656–669.)* All the drugs listed in the question are usually considered nonsteroidal anti-inflammatory drugs (NSAIDs), a large group of structurally dissimilar compounds. These drugs share the pharmacologic properties of the prototype compound, aspirin, in that all have analgesic, antipyretic, and anti-inflammatory effects. The mechanism of action responsible for these effects is reduction in the formation of eicosanoids (e.g., prostaglandins, thromboxanes) by inhibition of the enzyme cyclooxygenase. Drugs in this group are used to treat a variety of inflammatory conditions (e.g., rheumatoid arthritis, osteoarthritis) and pain. Acetaminophen differs from the other drugs in that it is a very weak anti-inflammatory agent and is not useful for treating inflammatory diseases. This drug is an effective analgesic and antipyretic; therefore, it is indicated for the reduction of pain and fever.

359. The answer is E. *(DiPalma, 4/e, pp 199–201. Katzung, 6/e, pp 262–264.)* In the periphery, serotonin, known chemically as *5-hydroxytryptamine (5-HT)*, exerts many effects on a variety of tissues. The effects of this endogenous amine are mediated through an array of 5-HT receptor subtypes and are species-dependent and variable, making it difficult to generalize. However, in humans all the effects described in the question may occur following exogenous administration of this substance except for relaxation of gastrointestinal smooth muscle. The enterochromaffin cells of the intestine contain about 90 percent of the body's stores of 5-HT. The amine causes gastrointestinal smooth muscle to contract by both a direct action on 5-HT receptors of the muscle and by stimulation of parasympathetic ganglia found within the intestinal wall. Although it is believed that 5-HT serves a physiologic function by increasing tone and facilitating peristalsis, it may also be involved in certain diseases, e.g., carcinoid tumor, in which an overproduction of 5-HT results in diarrhea.

Renal System

Carbonic Anhydrase Inhibitors
  Acetazolamide*
Loop Diuretics
  Bumetanide
  Ethacrynic acid
  Furosemide*
  Torsemide
Osmotic Diuretics
  Mannitol
Potassium-Sparing Diuretics
  Amiloride
  Spironolactone*
  Trimaterene*

Thiazide Diuretics
  Bendroflumethiazide
  Chlorothiazide*
  Hydrochlorothiazide
  Polythiazide
Thiazide-Related Compounds
  Chlorthalidone
  Indapamide
  Metolazone
Antidiuretic Hormone
  Vasopressin*
  Desmopressin
  Lypressin

DIRECTIONS: Each question below contains five suggested responses. Select the **one best** response to each question.

360. The structure shown below is a member of which of the following drug groups?

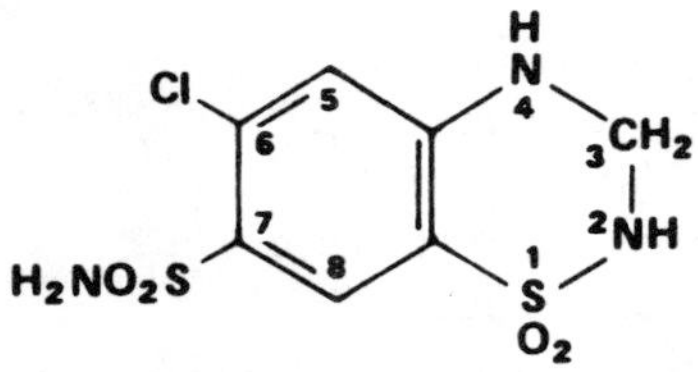

(A) Osmotic diuretics
(B) Loop diuretics
(C) Thiazide diuretics
(D) Potassium-sparing diuretics
(E) Carbonic anhydrase inhibitors

361. Torsemide (Demadex) inhibits the Na^+-K^+-$2Cl^-$ cotransporters that are located in the

(A) collecting duct
(B) ascending limb of the loop of Henle
(D) descending limb of the loop of Henle
(D) proximal tubule
(E) distal involuted tubule

362. Canrenone, which elicits a diuretic response, is a major biotransformation product of which of the following agents?

(A) Indapamide (Lozol)
(B) Chlorthalidone (Hygroton)
(C) Spironolactone (Aldactone)
(D) Amiloride (Midamor)
(E) Triamterene (Dyrenium)

363. Hyperkalemia is a contraindication to the use of which of the following drugs?

(A) Acetazolamide (Diamox)
(B) Chlorothiazide (Diuril)
(C) Ethacrynic acid (Edecrin)
(D) Chlorthalidone (Hygroton)
(E) Spironolactone (Aldactone)

364. A reduction in insulin release from the pancreas may be caused by which of the following diuretics?

(A) Triamterene (Dyrenium)
(B) Chlorothiazide (Diuril)
(C) Spironolactone (Aldactone)
(D) Acetazolamide (Diamox)
(E) Amiloride (Midamor)

365. Acute uric acid nephropathy, which is characterized by the acute overproduction of uric acid and by extreme hyperuricemia, can best be prevented with

(A) antidiuretic hormone (vasopressin, ADH)
(B) cyclophosphamide (Cytoxan)
(C) allopurinol (Zyloprim)
(D) amiloride (Midamor)
(E) sodium chloride

366. Idiopathic calcium urolithiasis can be treated by the administration of

(A) ethacrynic acid (Edecrin)
(B) triamterene (Dyrenium)
(C) furosemide (Lasix)
(D) hydrochlorothiazide (Hydrodiuril)
(E) bumetanide (Bumex)

367. A hospitalized patient, who has been maintained on parenteral alimentation for 3 weeks, develops weakness, tremors, agitation, and finally coma. The most likely fluid and electrolyte disturbance is

(A) hyperkalemia
(B) dehydration
(C) hypomagnesemia
(D) acidosis
(E) hypercalcemia

368. The release of antidiuretic hormone (ADH) is suppressed by which of the following drugs to promote a diuresis?

(A) Guanethidine (Ismelin)
(B) Acetazolamide (Diamox)
(C) Chlorothiazide (Diuril)
(D) Ethanol
(E) Indomethacin (Indocin)

369. Antidiuretic hormone (vasopressin) is used therapeutically for

(A) increasing uterine contractility
(B) treating nephrogenic diabetes insipidus
(C) treating pituitary diabetes insipidus
(D) treating polyuria caused by hypercalcemia
(E) decreasing chest pain in refractory unstable angina

370. Conservation of potassium ions in the body occurs with which of the following diuretics?

(A) Furosemide (Lasix)
(B) Hydrochlorothiazide (Hydrodiuril)
(C) Triamterene (Dyrenium)
(D) Metolazone (Zaroxolyn)
(E) Bumetanide (Bumex)

371. Spironolactone (Aldactone) can be characterized by which one of the following statements?

(A) It is biotransformed to an inactive product
(B) It binds to a cytoplasmic receptor
(C) It is a more potent diuretic than is hydrochlorothiazide
(D) It interferes with aldosterone synthesis
(E) It inhibits sodium reabsorption in the proximal renal tubule of the nephron

372. The distal tubule of the nephron is the principal site of action for which one of the following?

(A) Bumetanide (Bumex)
(B) Hydrochlorothiazide (Hydrodiuril)
(C) Ethacrynic acid (Edecrin)
(D) Triamterene (Dyrenium)
(E) Amiloride (Midamor)

373. Which of the following agents causes a reduction in the hypertonicity of the medullary interstitium of the kidney?

(A) Metolazone (Zaroxolyn)
(B) Spironolactone (Aldactone)
(C) Hydrochlorothiazide (Hydrodiuril)
(D) Mannitol
(E) Ethacrynic acid (Edecrin)

374. An enhancement of the parathyroid hormone–mediated reabsorption of calcium in the distal tubule is caused by which of the following diuretics?

(A) Acetazolamide (Diamox)
(B) Furosemide (Lasix)
(C) Triamterene (Dyrenium)
(D) Bumetanide (Bumex)
(E) Hydrochlorothiazide (Hydrodiuril)

DIRECTIONS: Each numbered question or incomplete statement below is NEGATIVELY phrased. Select the **one best** lettered response.

375. Mannitol may be useful in all the following procedures EXCEPT

(A) treatment of elevated intracranial pressure
(B) treatment of elevated intraocular pressure
(C) treatment of pulmonary edema with congestive heart failure
(D) diagnostic evaluation of acute oliguria
(E) prophylaxis of acute renal failure

376. When furosemide (Lasix) is administered concomitantly with other drugs, all the following can occur EXCEPT

(A) reduction of renal clearance of lithium
(B) enhancement of ototoxicity of gentamicin
(C) reduction of renal excretion of salicylates
(D) augmentation of pressor action of norepinephrine
(E) attenuation of neuromuscular blocking effect of tubocurarine

377. Adverse interactions may occur between thiazides and all the following drug groups EXCEPT

(A) adrenal corticosteroids
(B) anticoagulants (oral)
(C) aminoglycosides
(D) beta-adrenergic blockers
(E) antidepolarizing skeletal muscle relaxants

378. Diuretic agents that indirectly cause an increased binding of digoxin to cardiac tissue Na^+,K^+-ATPase include all the following EXCEPT

(A) hydrochlorothiazide (Hydrodiuril)
(B) torsemide (Demadex)
(C) amiloride (Midamor)
(D) ethacrynic acid (Edecrin)
(E) indapamide (Lozol)

379. Properties of mannitol include all the following EXCEPT

(A) retention of water in the tubular fluid
(B) the ability to be metabolically altered to an active form
(C) the capacity to be freely filtered
(D) effectiveness as nonelectrolytic, osmotically active particles
(E) the ability to resist complete reabsorption by the renal tubule

380. True statements about adverse reactions that apply to *both* hydrochlorothiazide (Hydrodiuril) and torsemide (Demadex) include all the following EXCEPT

(A) they may produce hyperglycemia
(B) they elevate blood levels of uric acid
(C) they decrease blood pressure
(D) they may cause hyperlipidemia
(E) they lower serum levels of magnesium

381. Adverse reactions associated with furosemide (Lasix) include all the following EXCEPT

(A) hyperglycemia
(B) tinnitus
(C) fluid and electrolyte imbalance
(D) hypotension
(E) metabolic acidosis

382. Chlorothiazide increases the urinary excretion of all the following ions EXCEPT

(A) potassium
(B) chloride
(C) calcium
(D) sodium
(E) magnesium

383. Correct statements regarding amiloride (Midamor) include all the following EXCEPT

(A) it carries an increased risk of hyperkalemia when given with an ACE inhibitor
(B) it is used in combination with furosemide
(C) it exhibits mild diuretic activity
(D) it inhibits sodium reabsorption
(E) it is a prodrug

384. Adverse reactions associated with both acetazolamide (Diamox) and antibacterial sulfonamides include all the following EXCEPT

(A) formation of urinary calculi
(B) fever
(C) metabolic acidosis
(D) crystalluria
(E) exfoliative dermatitis

385. Hydrochlorothiazide is clinically useful in the treatment of all the following EXCEPT

(A) edema caused by congestive heart failure
(B) edema induced by glucocorticoids
(C) hypertension with or without edema
(D) liver disease with ascites
(E) glaucoma by reduction of intraocular pressure

DIRECTIONS: Each group of questions below consists of lettered headings followed by a set of numbered items. For each numbered item select the **one** lettered heading with which it is **most** closely associated. Each lettered heading may be used **once, more than once, or not at all.**

Questions 386–388

The figure below shows proposed sites of action of drugs. For each of the diuretic agents below, choose the anatomic site in the schematic diagram of the renal nephron where the principal action of the agent occurs.

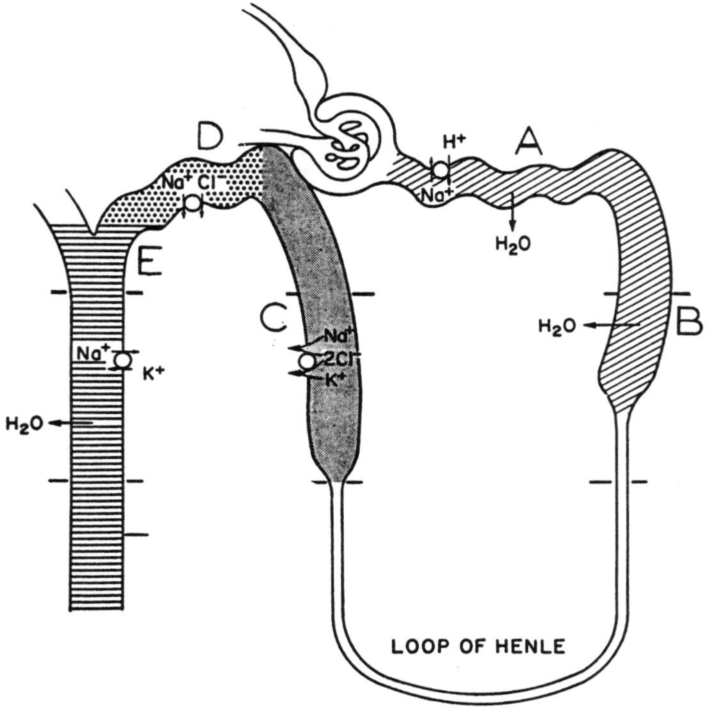

(Modified from DiPalma, 4/e, with permission.)

386. Ethacrynic acid (Edecrin)

387. Indapamide (Lozol)

388. Triamterene (Dyrenium)

Questions 389–391

The table below shows the urinary excretion patterns of electrolytes of diuretic drugs. For each of the diuretic agents listed below, choose the urinary excretion pattern that the drug would produce.

Drug	Na^+	Cl^-	K^+	Ca^{2+}	HCO_3^-	Mg^{2+}
(A)	+	+	+	−	±	+
(B)	+	+	+	−	0	+
(C)	+	+	+	+	0	+
(D)	+	+	−	0	+	0
(E)	+	−	+	0	+	0

+ = increase; − = decrease; 0 = no change; ± = increase dependent on dose

389. Triamterene (Dyrenium)

390. Torsemide

391. Bumetanide (Bumex)

Questions 392–394

Match each statement with the appropriate drug.

(A) Metolazone (Zaroxolyn)
(B) Ethacrynic acid (Edecrin)
(C) Chlorthalidone (Hygroton)
(D) Triamterene (Dyrenium)
(E) Spironolactone (Aldactone)
(F) Acetazolamide (Diamox)
(G) Furosemide (Lasix)
(H) Mannitol
(I) Amiloride (Midamor)
(J) Hydrochlorothiazide

392. The urinary excretion of chloride is decreased

393. Elevated intraocular and cerebrospinal fluid pressures are reduced

394. Chemically, this compound is a steroid

Renal System
Answers

360. The answer is C. *(DiPalma, 4/e, pp 457–458, 463–464. Gilman, 8/e, p 720.)* The structure shown in the question is hydrochlorothiazide (Esidrix) and is one of several of the thiazide (benzothiadiazide) diuretics. Halogenation of the benzothiadiazine ring at C 6 and a free sulfamyl group (—SO_2NH_2) at C 7 are necessary for maximal diuretic activity in the series of compounds. In contrast to the carbonic anhydrase inhibitors, benzothiadiazides can act independently of acid-base balance. An example of an osmotic diuretic is mannitol; representatives of the loop diuretics are furosemide, ethacrynic acid, and bumetanide. Potassium-sparing diuretics are spironolactone (a steroid), triamterene (a pyrazine derivative), and amiloride (a pyrazinecarbonyl-guanidine).

361. The answer is B. *(DiPalma, 4/e, pp 455–456, 460–462.)* Torsemide is a loop diuretic that promotes the urinary excretion of sodium and chloride. This diuretic agent blocks the reabsorption of sodium and chloride by inhibiting the Na^+-K^+-$2Cl^-$ cotransporters in the ascending limb of the loop of Henle. Although this cotransport mechanism requires energy from converting ATP to APP by Na^+,K^+-ATPase, torsemide does not directly inhibit the enzyme, Na^+,K^+-ATPase. Along with the net loss of sodium and chloride, loop diuretics produce an increase in the urinary excretion of calcium and magnesium by interfering with the reabsorption of these ions in the ascending limb of the loop of Henle. In addition, torsemide, like the other loop diuretic agents, can cause hypokalemia. The secretion of the potassium occurs as a consequence of the reabsorption of sodium in the late distal convoluted tubule and the collecting duct. The diuretic effect of torsemide has a duration of 6 to 8 h.

362. The answer is C. *(DiPalma, 4/e, pp 463–464. Gilman, 8/e, pp 725–728.)* Canrenone is the active biotransformation product of spironolactone. Similar to spironolactone, it is a competitive antagonist of aldosterone in the collecting duct of the nephron. Canrenone, like spironolactone, can bind to the cytoplasmic aldosterone receptor and prevent the receptor from being converted to the active conformation. Since the active conformation is prevented, reduction of sodium chloride reabsorption and potassium retention results. The diuretic action of spironolactone is partially due to the presence of canrenone. Indapamide, chlorthalidone, amiloride, and furosemide are not biotransformed to active products. Triamterene, however, is converted to some products that exhibit diuretic activity.

363. The answer is E. *(DiPalma, 4/e, pp 463–464. Gilman, 8/e, p 726.)* Spironolactone (Aldactone) is a competitive antagonist of aldosterone that blocks the reabsorption of sodium and water from the collecting duct in exchange for potassium and hydrogen ion retention. Therefore, in the presence of hyperkalemia, spironolactone is contraindicated. The administration of each of the other diuretic agents listed in the question results in increased excretion of potassium.

364. The answer is B. *(DiPalma, 4/e, pp 458–459, 461–462. Gilman, 8/e, p 721.)* An adverse reaction reported to occur occasionally with the thiazides, such as chlorothiazide, is hyperglycemia. In addition hyperglycemia may occur with thiazide-related compounds (chlorothalidone and metolazone) and the high-ceiling diuretics (ethacrynic acid, furosemide, and bumetanide). The proposed mechanism for the elevation in blood glucose appears to be related to a decrease in insulin release from the pancreas. In addition increased glycogenolysis, decreased glycogenesis, and a reduction in the conversion of proinsulin to insulin may also be involved in the hyperglycemic response. Diazoxide, a nondiuretic thiazide, is given to treat hypoglycemia in certain conditions. However, diazoxide is used more often to control hypertensive emergencies.

365. The answer is C. *(DiPalma, 4/e, pp 362–363, 660. Gilman, 8/e, p 678.)* Acute hyperuricemia, which often occurs in patients treated with cytotoxic drugs for neoplasic disorders, can lead to the deposition of urate crystals in the kidneys and their collecting ducts. This can produce partial or complete obstruction of the collecting ducts, renal pelvis, or ureter. Allopurinol and its primary metabolite, alloxanthine, are inhibitors of xanthine oxidase, an enzyme that catalyzes the oxidation of hypoxanthine and xanthine to uric acid. The use of allopurinol in patients at risk can markedly reduce the likelihood that they will develop acute uric acid nephropathy.

366. The answer is D. *(DiPalma, 4/e, pp 457, 460, 462. Katzung, 6/e, p 555.)* In the nephron unit calcium ions are reabsorbed from the renal tubular fluid in the cortical portion of the ascending limb of Henle and in the distal tubule. Parathyroid hormone mediates the transport of calcium in the distal tubule. Thiazide diuretics and thiazide-related compounds enhance the reabsorption of calcium ions in the distal tubule and therefore reduce urinary excretion of calcium. This effect of thiazide diuretics and related compounds makes these drugs useful in the treatment of idiopathic calcium urolithiasis.

The loop diuretics such as furosemide, bumetanide, torsemide, and ethacrynic acid tend to enhance the urinary excretion of calcium. They reduce the reabsorption of calcium in the ascending limb of the loop of Henle and, therefore, lower serum levels of calcium. These drugs are effective in the acute treatment of hypercalcemia.

367. The answer is C. *(Gilman, 8/e, p 705.)* Hypomagnesemia is characterized by signs and symptoms that usually include disturbances in the nervous and muscular systems, psychotic behavior, tetany, tachycardia, and hypertension. Because few parenteral alimentation fluids contain magnesium, the clinical manifestations of hypomagnesemia are most commonly found in association with the prolonged parenteral alimentation of magnesium-free solutions.

368. The answer is D. *(DiPalma, 4/e, pp 256, 457, 465. Gilman, 8/e, p 374.)* Ethanol produces a diuretic response by inhibiting the release of antidiuretic hormone (ADH) from the posterior pituitary gland. Less antidiuretic hormone acts on the collecting duct of the nephron and, therefore, the amount of water reabsorbed by the collecting duct is reduced. Indomethacin enhances the release of antidiuretic hormone, which increases the permeability of the collecting duct to water. Acetazolamide and chlorothiazide promote a diuresis by acting on site directly in the nephron unit to reduce the reabsorption of sodium chloride and water. Guanethidine, an antihypertensive agent, does not appear to alter the release of antidiuretic hormone.

369. The answer is C. *(Katzung, 6/e, pp 574–575.)* Small doses of antidiuretic hormone (vasopressin) or the newer synthetic analogue, desmopressin, can control polyuria and polydipsia in diabetes insipidus caused by pituitary insufficiency. Other syndromes that mimic the polyuria of vasopressin deficiency, such as nephrogenic diabetes insipidus and hypercalcemia, do not respond to antidiuretic hormone (vasopressin). Although antidiuretic hormone (vasopressin) has intrinsic oxytocic activity, it remains relatively ineffective for initiating or intensifying uterine contractions. Antidiuretic hormone is not used in the treatment of angina because the drug produces coronary vasoconstriction. The drug should be used with caution in patients with ischemic heart disease.

370. The answer is C. *(DiPalma, 4/e, pp 457–464. Gilman, 8/e, pp 721–728.)* Triamterene produces retention of the potassium ion by inhibiting in the collecting duct the reabsorption of sodium, which is accompanied by the excretion of potassium ions. The loop diuretics furosemide and bumetanide cause as a possible adverse action the development of hypokalemia. In addition, thiazides (e.g., hydrochlorothiazide) and the thiazide-related agents (e.g., metolazone) can cause the loss of potassium ions with the consequences of hypokalemia. Triamterene is generally given with a loop diuretic or thiazide to prevent or correct the condition of hypokalemia.

371. The answer is B. *(DiPalma, 4/e, pp 463–464. Gilman, 8/e, pp 725–726.)* Spironolactone is a potassium-sparing diuretic. The drug is well absorbed from the gastrointestinal tract and is biotransformed in the liver to an active metabolite, canrenone. Spironolactone is contraindicated in the presence of hyperkalemia, since this aldosterone antagonist may cause further elevation of plasma potassium concentrations. It does not appear to depress adrenal or pituitary function. CNS side effects of the drug can include lethargy, headache, drowsiness, and mental confusion. Spironolactone displaces aldosterone from receptor sites that are responsible for sodium resorption in the collecting duct of the nephron; it does not interfere with the synthesis of aldosterone.

372. The answer is B. *(DiPalma, 4/e, pp 457, 459–460, 463, 465. Katzung, 6/e, pp 237–242.)* Diuretic agents exert their effect to promote a net loss of sodium and water by blocking the reabsorption of sodium ions at various regions of the nephron unit. The thiazide diuretics (e.g., hydrochlorothiazide) and the thiazide-related compounds (chlorthalidone, metolazone, and indapamide) interfere with the reabsorption of sodium ions in the distal tubule. These diuretics cause an increase in urinary excretion of sodium, chloride, potassium, water, and, in the case of chlorothiazide, bicarbonate. The loop diuretics (e.g., bumetanide, ethacrynic acid, and furosemide) reduce the cotransport of sodium and chloride ions from the ascending limb of the loop of Henle. There occurs an increased urinary excretion of sodium, chloride, potassium, hydrogen, magnesium, and calcium. Since loop diuretics reduce the tonicity of the medullary interstitium, free-water reabsorption is decreased in the collecting duct. The potassium-sparing diuretics (spironolactone, triamterene, and amiloride) exert their diuretic action by blocking the reabsorption of sodium in the late distal tubule and collecting duct.

373. The answer is E. *(DiPalma, 4/e, pp 456–457, 460. Katzung, 6/e, pp 237–239.)* In the ascending limb of the loop of Henle it is the medullary portion of the ascending limb that participates in maintaining the hypertonicity of the interstitium by the cotransport of sodium and chloride from the renal tubular fluid. The medullary hypertonicity contributes to the concentration of urine. The loop diuretics (ethacrynic acid, furosemide, torsemide, and bumetanide) inhibit the cotransport of sodium and chloride in both the cortical and medullary portions of the ascending limb and reduce the medullary hypertonicity. As a consequence of this action, free-water reabsorption in the collecting duct of the nephron is reduced; therefore, increased amounts of sodium, chloride, and water are excreted from the body.

374. The answer is E. *(DiPalma, 4/e, pp 456–458, 460. Gilman, 8/e, pp 719, 722.)* In the distal tubule of the nephron sodium and chloride ions are reabsorbed. In addition, calcium ions are reabsorbed by a parathyroid-mediated response. Thiazide diuretics (e.g., hydrochlorothiazide) have their site of action on the distal tubule and inhibit the reabsorption of sodium and chloride but enhance the parathyroid-mediated increase of calcium reabsorption. The urinary excretion of sodium and chloride is increased, while excretion of calcium is reduced. Loop diuretics such as furosemide and bumetanide increase the urinary excretion of calcium ions and may be used in the treatment of acute hypercalcemia. Acetazolamide and triamterene do not appear to inhibit the reabsorption of calcium ions in the distal tubule.

375. The answer is C. *(DiPalma, 4/e, p 466. Gilman, 8/e, pp 714–715.)* Mannitol increases serum osmolarity and therefore "pulls" water out of cells, cerebrospinal fluid, and aqueous humor. This effect can be useful in the treatment of elevated intraocular or intracranial pressure. However, by expanding the intravascular volume, mannitol can exacerbate congestive heart failure. Mannitol will increase urine output if oliguria is caused by a decreased glomerular filtration rate but not if the oliguria is secondary to tubular dysfunction. Mannitol is useful in the prevention of acute renal failure as a means of maintaining an adequate flow of relatively dilute urine.

376. The answer is D. *(DiPalma, 4/e, p 462. Gilman, 8/e, p 724.)* The diuretic agents are involved in a number of interactions when they are given concomitantly with another drug. The loop diuretic furosemide is an example of this class of drugs that can cause several drug-drug interactions. Furosemide can enhance the toxicity of lithium by reducing its renal excretion. Since the loop diuretic can cause hearing impairment, it can augment the ototoxicity that can occur with other drugs, such as aminoglycoside antibiotics (e.g., gentamicin, streptomycin, tobramycin). Furosemide undergoes proximal tubule secretion. This renal secretory mechanism, which is associated with renal excretion, is also available to a number of organic acids, such as the salicylates. When salicylates are present in the body, furosemide is a competitive inhibitor of their excretion by this particular mechanism in the proximal tubule; therefore, the plasma levels of salicylates are increased with the potential for adverse reactions in the patient. Interactions between norepinephrine and furosemide have been reported. The hypertensive effect of norepinephrine is decreased when it is administered with furosemide. Furosemide should be discontinued in a patient prior to surgery. This diuretic agent may also reduce the skeletal muscle relaxant effects of tubocurarine.

377. The answer is C. *(AMA Drug Evaluations Annual, 1993, p 692. DiPalma, 4/e, pp 458–459.)* Drug interactions are reported for various drugs and the thiazide diuretics. Thiazides can indirectly promote the loss of potassium from the collecting duct of the nephron, and adrenal corticosteroids can enhance the hypokalemic effect. The therapeutic effect of oral anticoagulants may be reduced by thiazides because these diuretics can concentrate clotting factors in the blood. Thiazide diuretics elevate blood lipid, urate, and glucose levels and these effects can be augmented in the presence of a beta-adrenergic blocker. In addition, the neuromuscular blocking action of tubocurarine is enhanced by thiazide diuretics. Aminoglycosides, which can cause eighth nerve damage, can increase the ototoxicity that is associated with the use of the loop diuretics. Tinnitus and ototoxicity have not been reported as adverse reactions for the thiazide diuretics.

378. The answer is C. *(DiPalma, 4/e, pp 458, 461, 464. Gilman, 8/e, pp 701, 719, 722, 726.)* Diuretic therapy can lead to the development of hypokalemia. The thiazides (hydrochlorothiazide), thiazide-related compounds (indapamide), and loop diuretics (e.g., ethacrynic acid and torsemide) can produce the loss of potassium from the blood through the late distal tubule and collecting duct into the renal tubular fluid. When any of these drugs are administered in the presence of digitalis glycoside (digoxin), there is the potential for digitalis toxicities to occur. The development of these toxicities is related to the fact that in the presence of hypokalemia there is greater affinity of digitalis glycosides to cardiac tissue Na^+,K^+-ATPase. However, when the hypokalemia is corrected and the plasma levels of potassium are returned toward normal, digitalis toxicities are usually eliminated. Amiloride, which is a potassium-sparing diuretic, does not cause hypokalemia and, therefore, would not enhance the binding of digoxin to Na^+,K^+-ATPase. As a matter of fact, amiloride promotes the conservation of potassium and can cause the adverse reaction of hyperkalemia.

379. The answer is B. *(DiPalma, 4/e, p 466. Gilman, 8/e, pp 714–715.)* A significant increase in the amount of any osmotically active solute in voided urine is usually accompanied by an increase in urine volume. Osmotic diuretics effect diuresis through this principle. The osmotic diuretics (such as mannitol) are nonelectrolytes that are freely filtered at the glomerulus, undergo limited reabsorption by the renal tubules, retain water in the renal tubule, and promote an osmotic diuresis, generally without significant sodium excretion. In addition, these diuretics resist alteration by metabolic processes.

380. The answer is D. *(DiPalma, 4/e, pp 458, 461–462. Gilman, 8/e, pp 721, 723–724.)* The thiazide diuretics and the loop diuretics have a number of adverse reactions in common. Hydrochlorothiazide and the loop diuretic torsemide cause hyperglycemia by possibly reducing the secretion of insulin from the pancreas. Since these drugs can elevate blood levels of glucose they should be used with caution when administered to patients with diabetes mellitus. The development of hyperuricemia as a consequence of the use of hydrochlorothiazide or torsemide is related to the fact that these drugs interfere with the proximal tubule secretion of uric acid and cause volume depletion. Neither torsemide nor hydrochlorothiazide has any effect on the synthesis of uric acid. Both hydrochlorothiazide and torsemide are indicated in the treatment of hypertension. These drugs will bring about a reduction in elevated blood pressure. This effect is considered an adverse reaction if it occurs when the drugs are employed as diuretic agents to remove edematous fluid from a patient. Of the diuretic agents only the thiazide drugs have been reported to cause an elevation in blood lipids (hyperlipidemia). The mechanism of action for this effect on lipids is unknown. The alteration in serum magnesium (hypomagnesemia) is caused by both hydrochlorothiazide and torsemide. These diuretic agents block the reabsorption of magnesium.

381. The answer is E. *(DiPalma, 4/e, pp 460–462. Gilman, 8/e, pp 723–724.)* The loop, or high-ceiling, diuretics furosemide and ethacrynic acid are cleared by the kidney with such celerity that even high doses repeatedly administered do not result in significant accumulation. Chronic administration of these agents, however, may lead to alkalosis with hyponatremia in association with rapid removal of edema fluid. Other toxic manifestations of loop diuretics include fluid and electrolyte imbalance, gastrointestinal symptoms, interstitial nephritis, hyperglycemia, tinnitus, and infrequent, but serious, ototoxicity. Besides being used as a diuretic agent, furosemide is used in the treatment of hypertension.

382. The answer is C. *(DiPalma, 4/e, pp 457–458. Gilman, 8/e, pp 718–719.)* Thiazide diuretics enhance the excretion of sodium, chloride, potassium, and magnesium ions. The excretion of calcium appears to be reduced following chronic drug administration. Since the thiazide diuretics inhibit sodium chloride reabsorption in the early portion of the distal tubule, an increased load of sodium and chloride ions is presented to the collecting duct. In this region some sodium ions may be actively reabsorbed and potassium ions secreted, which leads to an increased loss of potassium from the body.

383. The answer is E. *(AMA Drug Evaluations Annual, 1993, p 809. DiPalma, 4/e, pp 463–465.)* Amiloride is a potassium-sparing diuretic with a mild diuretic and natriuretic effect. The parent compound is active and the drug is excreted unchanged in the urine. Amiloride has a duration of action of 24 h and is usually administered with a thiazide or loop diuretic (e.g., furosemide) to prevent the development of hypokalemia. The site of the diuretic action of amiloride is the late distal tubule and collecting duct, where it interferes with the reabsorption of sodium and allows for the retention of potassium. The drug is contraindicated in hyperkalemia. In addition, it has been reported that there is an increased risk of hyperkalemia when an ACE inhibitor is used with amiloride or spironolactone.

384. The answer is C. *(DiPalma, 4/e, p 465. Katzung, 6/e, pp 234–236.)* Acetazolamide, an aromatic sulfonamide derivative, is a mild diuretic agent that increases the loss of sodium and water from the body by inhibiting the enzyme carbonic anhydrase. The sulfonamides, a group of antibacterial agents, exert their antimicrobial effect on gram-positive and gram-negative bacteria by competitive antagonism of para-aminobenzoic acid (PABA). Acetazolamide and the sulfonamides are reported to have some similar adverse reactions. Fever, blood dyscrasias, exfoliative dermatitis, skin rash, crystalluria, and formation of calculi may occur with the administration of either. Metabolic acidosis is associated only with the use of acetazolamide. Since this diuretic inhibits carbonic anhydrase in the proximal tubule, plasma levels of bicarbonate decrease, and if the reduction of bicarbonate is significant, metabolic acidosis can develop.

385. The answer is E. *(DiPalma, 4/e, pp 459, 465. Gilman, 8/e, p 721.)* Thiazides are most useful as diuretic agents in the management of edema caused by chronic cardiac decompensation. In the treatment of hypertensive disease, even without obvious edema, thiazides exert a hypotensive action that has proved beneficial. Less common uses of thiazide diuretics include the treatment of edema from glucocorticoids, diabetes insipidus, and hypercalciuria. The carbonic anhydrase inhibitor acetazolamide (Diamox), by inhibiting the secretion of aqueous humor, has the property of decreasing intraocular pressure—an effect of value for patients who have glaucoma. Furosemide is the diuretic agent generally employed to treat acute pulmonary edema, although ethacrynic acid would be effective.

386–388. The answers are 386-C, 387-D, 388-E. *(DiPalma, 4/e, pp 456–466. Gilman, 8/e, pp 718, 722, 725–727.)* The loop diuretic ethacrynic acid has its site of action in the ascending limb of the loop of Henle. This drug inhibits the reabsorption of sodium and chloride by interfering with the Na^+-K^+-$2Cl^-$ cotransport system. In addition, loop diuretics block the reabsorption of magnesium and calcium from the renal tubular fluid into the blood in this segment of the nephron unit.

Indapamide, which is a thiazide-related compound, has its proposed site of action at the distal convoluted tubule or more specifically at the early portion of the distal tubule. The distal convoluted tubule is also the site of action for the thiazide diuretic agents (e.g., chlorothiazide and hydrochlorothiazide). Indapamide and hydrochlorothiazide inhibit the reabsorption of sodium and chloride. These diuretics also promote the reabsorption of calcium back into the blood, but inhibit the reabsorption of magnesium from the renal tubular fluid.

The potassium-sparing diuretic agents (spironolactone, triamterene, and amiloride) have their site of action in the nephron at the late distal tubule and the collecting duct. These diuretic agents only cause a mild natriuretic effect.

389–391. The answers are 389-D, 390-C, 391-C. *(DiPalma, 4/e, pp 457, 458, 460, 463–466. Gilman, 8/e, p 717.)* The urinary excretion pattern of electrolytes for the thiazide diuretic agents (e.g., chlorothiazide) is represented by choice A. These drugs block the reabsorption of sodium and chloride at the early distal convoluted tubule of the nephron. In addition, they promote the excretion of potassium and magnesium. At high doses the thiazide diuretics (especially chlorothiazide) may cause a slight increase in bicarbonate excretion. As for the calcium ion, the thiazide diuretic agents enhance the distal tubular reabsorption of calcium, and, therefore, calcium urinary excretion may decrease.

The thiazide-related compounds (e.g., chlorthalidone, metolazone, and indapamide) cause the same urinary excretion pattern of electrolytes but do not produce any change in bicarbonate excretion, since these drugs do not have the ability to inhibit carbonic anhydrase. The thiazide-related drugs are represented by choice B.

The loop diuretics (e.g., torsemide, bumetanide, furosemide, and ethacrynic acid) are the most potent group of diuretic agents, and they are represented by choice C in the table. These drugs act at the ascending limb of the loop of Henle and interfere with the cotransport of sodium and chloride. In addition, they cause the excretion of potassium, magnesium, and calcium into the urine.

The potassium-sparing group of diuretic agents are represented by choice D in the table. Triamterene produces its diuretic response by reduction of the reabsorption of sodium in the later distal convoluted tubule and the collecting duct. It causes an increase in the urinary excretion of sodium chloride and possibly bicarbonate, while it reduces the excretion of potassium. The potassium-sparing diuretic agents do not appear to have any significant effect on the excretion of magnesium and calcium ions.

392–394. The answers are 392-F, 393-H, 394-E. *(DiPalma, 4/e, pp 463, 465–466. Gilman, 8/e, pp 715, 725–726.)* Acetazolamide is a carbonic anhydrase inhibitor with its primary site of action at the proximal tubule of the nephron. Acetazolamide promotes a urinary excretion of sodium, potassium, and bicarbonate. There is a decrease in loss of chloride ions. The increased excretion of bicarbonate makes the urine alkaline and may produce metabolic acidosis as a consequence of the loss of bicarbonate from the blood. None of the other diuretic drugs promote a reduction in the excretion of the chloride ion.

The only diuretic agent that has a steroid structure is spironolactone. This potassium-sparing diuretic is a competitive inhibitor of aldosterone, which mediates the reabsorption of sodium ions in the collecting duct.

Mannitol is classified as an osmotic diuretic. It is used to maintain urine flow in such cases as trauma and drug intoxication as well as after surgery. In addition, mannitol is used to reduce pressure and volume of cerebrospinal fluid and pre- and postoperatively for short-term reduction of intraocular pressure. Although acetazolamide is used in the treatment of glaucoma, it is not employed to decrease cerebrospinal fluid pressure.

Gastrointestinal System and Nutrition

- Antacids
  - Sodium bicarbonate
  - Aluminum hydroxide
  - Magnesium hydroxide
  - Calcium carbonate
- H_2-Receptor Antagonists
  - Cimetidine
  - Ranitidine
  - Famotidine
  - Nizatidine
- Proton-Pump Inhibitors
  - Omeprazole (Losec)
- Mucosal Protective Agents
  - Sucralfate
  - Colloidal bismuth compounds—Bismuth subsalicylate (Pepto-Bismol)
  - Prostaglandins—misoprostal (Cytotec)
- Promotion of GI Motility
  - Metoclopramide (Reglan)
  - Bethanechol
  - Cisapride (Propulsid)
- Pancreatic Replacement Enzymes
  - Pancrelipase (Pancrease, Cotazyme)
- Laxatives
  - Castor oil
  - Cascara, senna, aloes, phenolphthalein, bisacodyl
  - Stool softeners
    - Mineral oil, glycerine suppositories, dioctyl sodium sulfosuccinate (docusate)
  - Bulk laxatives
    - Hydrophilic colloids
    - Saline cathartics
- Antidiarrheal Drugs
  - Diphenoxylate, loperamide
- Dissolution of Gallstones
  - Chenodeoxycholic acid
  - Ursodiol (ursodeoxycholic acid)
- Chronic Inflammatory Bowel Disease
  - Sulfasalazine
- Portal System Encephalopathy
  - Lactulose
  - Branched-chain amino acids
- Vitamins
  - Water-soluble
    - Thiamine (B_1)
    - Riboflavin (B_2)
    - Nicotinic acid (niacin)
    - Pyridoxine (B_6)
    - Vitamin C (ascorbic acid)
    - Vitamin B_{12}
    - Folic acid
  - Fat-Soluble
    - Vitamin A
    - Vitamin D
    - Vitamin E
    - Vitamin K
  - Concept of recommended daily allowances

DIRECTIONS: Each question below contains five suggested responses. Select the **one best** response to each question.

395. Cimetidine slows the metabolism of many drugs because it inhibits the activity of

(A) monoamine oxidase
(B) cytochrome P-450
(C) tyrosine kinase
(D) H^+,K^+-ATPase
(E) phase II glucoronidation reactions

396. The absorption of phosphate is reduced when large and prolonged doses of which of the following antacids are given?

(A) Sodium bicarbonate
(B) Magnesium hydroxide
(C) Magnesium trisilicate
(D) Calcium carbonate
(E) Sucralfate

397. Omeprazole (Losec), a new agent for the promotion of healing of peptic ulcers, has a mechanism of action based on

(A) prostaglandins
(B) gastric secretion
(C) pepsin secretion
(D) H^+, K^+-ATPase
(E) anticholinergic action

398. An effective antidiarrheal agent that inhibits peristaltic movement is

(A) clonidine
(B) bismuth subsalicylate
(C) oral electrolyte solution
(D) atropine
(E) diphenoxylate

399. The approved indication for misoprostal (Cytotec) is

(A) reflux esophagitis
(B) healing of gastric ulcer
(C) healing of duodenal ulcer
(D) prevention of gastric ulceration in patients using large doses of aspirin-like drugs
(E) pathologic hypersecretory conditions such as Zollinger-Ellison syndrome

400. Metoclopramide (Reglan) has antiemetic properties because it

(A) accelerates gastric emptying time
(B) lowers esophageal sphincter pressure
(C) is a CNS dopamine receptor antagonist
(D) has cholinomimetic properties
(E) has sedative properties

401. The steatorrhea of pancreatic insufficiency can best be treated by

(A) cimetidine
(B) misoprostal
(C) bile salts
(D) pancrelipase
(E) secretin

402. Cholesterol gallstones may be dissolved by oral treatment with

(A) lovastatin
(B) dehydrocholic acid
(C) methyl tertiary butyl ether
(D) chenodeoxycholic acid
(E) monoctanoin

403. A drug of choice in the therapy of inflammatory bowel disease is

(A) sulfadiazine
(B) sulfasalazine
(C) sulfapyridine
(D) sulfamethoxazole
(E) salicylate sodium

404. An important drug in the therapy of portal systemic encephalopathy is

(A) lactulose
(B) lactate
(C) loperamide
(D) lorazepam
(E) loxapine

405. Bismuth salts are thought to be effective in peptic ulcer disease because they have bactericidal properties against

(A) *Escherichia coli*
(B) *Bacteroides fragilis*
(C) *Clostridium difficile*
(D) *Helicobacter pylori*
(E) *Staphylococcus aureus*

406. Misoprostol has a cytoprotective action on the gastrointestinal mucosa because it

(A) enhances secretion of mucus and bicarbonate ion
(B) neutralizes acid secretion
(C) antagonizes NSAIDs
(D) relieves ulcer symptoms
(E) coats the mucosa

407. For the severe form of nodulocystic acne vulgaris, the first line of therapy is the systemic use of

(A) vitamin A
(B) retinol
(C) tetracycline
(D) isotretinoin (13-*cis*-retinoic acid)
(E) ciprofloxacin

408. The primary pharmacologic action of omeprazole (Losec) is reduction of

(A) volume of gastric juice
(B) gastric motility
(C) secretion of pepsin
(D) secretion of gastric acid
(E) secretion of intrinsic factor

409. Which of the following vitamins in large doses is teratogenic?

(A) Vitamin A
(B) Vitamin B_{12}
(C) Vitamin C
(D) Vitamin D
(E) Vitamin E

410. Fat-soluble vitamins have generally a greater potential toxicity compared with water-soluble vitamins because they are

(A) more essential to vital metabolic processes
(B) metabolically faster
(C) avidly stored by the body
(D) administered in larger doses
(E) involved in more essential metabolic pathways

411. In the United States the "Recommended Daily Allowances" (RDAs) are periodically developed by the

(A) National Research Council
(B) Food and Drug Administration
(C) Department of Agriculture
(D) Department of Commerce
(E) Surgeon General

412. Which vitamin needs to be given in supplemental doses in order to prevent deficiency when a patient is given prolonged administration of isoniazid?

(A) Vitamin A
(B) Vitamin K
(C) Vitamin C
(D) Thiamine
(E) Pyridoxine

DIRECTIONS: Each numbered question or incomplete statement below is NEGATIVELY phrased. Select the **one best** lettered response.

413. Which of the following is a stool softener that does NOT decrease absorption of fat-soluble vitamins?

(A) Mineral oil
(B) Castor oil
(C) Docusate sodium (Colace)
(D) Phenolphthalein
(E) Cascara sagrada

414. True statements concerning sucralfate include all the following EXCEPT

(A) it contains polyaluminum hydroxide
(B) it maintains gel-like qualities even at acid pH
(C) it binds to ulcer craters more than to normal mucosa
(D) it has moderate acid-neutralizing properties
(E) it reacts very little with mucin

DIRECTIONS: Each group of questions below consists of lettered headings followed by a set of numbered items. For each numbered item select the **one** lettered heading with which it is **most** closely associated. Each lettered heading may be used **once, more than once, or not at all.**

Questions 415–416

Match each vitamin with the appropriate description.

(A) Excess amounts should be avoided when the patient is on levodopa
(B) Overdosage may lead to a psychotic state
(C) Improvement of vision especially in daylight might be attributable to this vitamin
(D) This vitamin is usually not included in the popular "one-a-day" vitamin preparations
(E) Retinoic acid is the natural form
(F) Acute intoxication with this vitamin causes hypertension, nausea and vomiting, and signs of increased CSF pressure
(G) This vitamin has hormonal functions
(H) This fat-soluble vitamin has mainly antioxidant properties
(I) In its water-soluble form, this fat-soluble vitamin is capable of producing kernicterus

415. Calcitriol

416. Menadione

Questions 417–418

For each vitamin, match the appropriate use or deficiency.

(A) Large doses are used to treat hyperlipoproteinemia
(B) Large doses are used to acidify urine
(C) This vitamin is used in the therapy of Wernicke's syndrome
(D) Large doses are used to cure psychosis
(E) Deficiency can cause angular stomatitis
(F) Deficiency can cause the common cold
(G) Deficiency can cause convulsions in children

417. Nicotinic acid

418. Thiamine

Questions 419–420

Match the main therapeutic potential with the correct listed gastrointestinal drug.

(A) Ranitidine
(B) Metronidazole
(C) Omeprazole
(D) Sucralfate
(E) Misoprostol
(F) Calcium carbonate
(G) Loperamide

419. Preferred drug therapy for Zollinger-Ellison syndrome

420. Helpful in selected cases of diarrhea

Questions 421–422

There are different mechanisms by which laxatives achieve their effects. Match the mechanism to the correct drug.

(A) Magnesium sulfate
(B) Methylcellulose
(C) Phenolphthalein
(D) Castor oil
(E) Lactulose
(F) Mineral oil
(G) Docusate sodium (dioctyl sodium sulfosuccinate)

421. Has a hyperosmotic mechanism different from that of saline cathartics

422. Increases colonic peristalsis and enhances fluid and electrolyte secretion into the bowel

Questions 423–424

A large number of endogenous and exogenous agents act to alter the rate of secretion of acid by the parietal cell. Match the mechanism to the agent.

(A) Histamine
(B) Prostaglandin
(C) Gastrin
(D) Acetylcholine
(E) Aspirin
(F) Propantheline
(G) Food
(H) Aluminum hydroxide
(I) Bismuth subsalicylate
(J) Omeprazole
(K) Misoprostol
(L) Sucralfate

423. Lowers gastric acidity by competitive antagonism of acetylcholine

424. Increases gastric acidity by preventing the action of inhibitory G protein on adenylate cylase

Gastrointestinal System and Nutrition

Answers

395. The answer is B. *(DiPalma, 4/e, pp 199, 562. Gilman, 8/e, p 901.)* Cimetidine reversibly inhibits cytochrome P-450. This is important in phase I biotransformation reactions and inhibits the metabolism of such drugs as warfarin, phenytoin, propranolol, metoprolol, quinidine, and theophylline. None of the other enzymes are significantly affected.

396. The answer is D. *(DiPalma, 4/e, p 568. Gilman, 8/e, p 9.)* Although aluminum hydroxide is generally considered to be the antacid that inhibits phosphate absorption, calcium carbonate is equally capable of this effect. This adverse effect may be hazardous in the presence of renal impairment.

397. The answer is D. *(DiPalma, 4/e, pp 862–863. Gilman, 8/e, pp 902–904.)* Omeprazole inhibits H^+,K^+-ATPase, which effectively stops the proton pump and thus prevents the formation of gastric acid. It is the most effective agent in severe cases of ulceration and esophageal reflux.

398. The answer is E. *(DiPalma, 4/e, p 570. Gilman, 8/e, pp 924–925.)* Diphenoxylate is a piperidine opioid related to meperidine. It inhibits peristalsis and hence increases the passage time of the intestinal bolus. It is combined with atropine to discourage use as a street drug. Atropine has little effect on peristalsis. Clonidine, bismuth subsalicylate, and rehydration therapy are all useful in some types of diarrhea, but none of them inhibit peristalsis.

399. The answer is D. *(DiPalma, 4/e, pp 564–565. Gilman, 8/e, p 911.)* Misoprostal is a prostaglandin E analogue that has antisecretory and mucosal protection properties in the stomach. Experimentally it protects against mucosal damage from NSAIDs, alcohol, and other toxic agents. It will also tend to heal existing ulcers but is inferior to other agents in this regard.

400. The answer is C. *(DiPalma, 4/e, pp 574–575. Gilman, 8/e, pp 926–928.)* Metoclopramide antagonizes the emetic effect of apomorphine, which is mediated by a dopamine receptor in the CNS. It also raises the lower esophageal sphincter pressure and relaxes the pyloric sphincter, which hastens gastric emptying time. This makes it useful in the therapy of reflux esophagitis.

401. The answer is D. *(Gilman, 8/e, pp 929–930. Isselbacher, 13/e, p 1530.)* Pancrelipase (Pancrease, Cotazym) is an alcoholic extract of hog pancreas that contains lipase, trypsin, and amylase. It is effective in reducing the steatorrhea of pancreatic insufficiency. None of the other drugs mentioned have significant action in the digestion of fats.

402. The answer is D. *(Gilman, 8/e, pp 930–931. Isselbacher, 13/e, p 1509.)* Chenodeoxycholic acid (chenodiol) and ursodiol have proved to be effective in some patients with cholesterol gallstones. Lovastatin lowers blood cholesterol levels but has no effect on gallstones. Methyl tertiary butyl ether and a new agent, monoctanoin, are infused directly into the common duct and will dissolve gallstones.

403. The answer is B. *(DiPalma, 4/e, p 577. Gilman, 8/e, p 1051.)* Sulfasalazine consists of sulfapyridine with 5-aminosalicylic acid linked by an azo bond. This bond is broken by bacteria that release the salicylic acid, which is believed to be the active agent. Sulfa drugs or salicylic acid used alone is not as effective. The mechanism of action is unknown but is believed to be protective action on the mucosa by inhibition of the synthesis of prostaglandins and leukotrienes.

404. The answer is A. *(DiPalma, 4/e, p 573. Gilman, 8/e, pp 919–920.)* Lactulose is a synthetic disaccharide (galactose-fructose) that is not absorbed. In moderate doses it acts as a laxative. In higher doses it is capable of binding ammonia and other toxins that form in the intestine in severe liver deficiency and that are believed to cause the encephalopathy. Loperamide is an antidiarrheal opioid; lorazepam is a CNS depressant; loxapine is a tricyclic antipsychotic.

405. The answer is D. *(DiPalma, 4/e, p 566. Isselbacher, 13/e, p 1367.)* It is now recognized that infection with *Helicobacter pylori* is a major etiologic factor in peptic ulcer disease. Bismuth salts are bactericidal for many organisms but especially for spirochetes. Colloidal bismuth salts such as bismuth subsalicylate also have a coating or cytoprotective action.

406. The answer is A. *(DiPalma, 4/e, pp 564–565. Gilman, 8/e, pp 611, 911.)* Misoprostol is a prostaglandin analogue of PGE with an affinity for the gastric mucosa. It stimulates the secretion of mucus and bicarbonate, enhances cell proliferation, preserves the microcirculation, and stabilizes tissue lysosomes. Misoprostol is approved by the FDA for protection against the ulcerogenic action of NSAIDs (not because it antagonizes NSAIDs).

407. The answer is D. *(DiPalma, 4/e, p 543. Gilman, 8/e, p 1561.)* Isotretinoin is actually a form of high-dose vitamin A therapy. Vitamin A itself or retinol (vitamin A_1) could be used, but they have less advantageous pharmacokinetic properties. Antibiotics such as tetracyclines are used in acne but have little effect on the nodulocystic form.

408. The answer is D. *(DiPalma, 4/e, pp 562–563. Gilman, 8/e, p 903.)* The main action of omeprazole is inhibition of secretion of gastric acid. Because it is a specific inhibitor of the proton pump (H^+,K^+-ATPase), other actions are secondary to the marked decline of acid secretion. As a result of the reduction of gastric acidity, there is increased secretion of gastrin leading to hypergastrinemia.

409. The answer is A. *(DiPalma, 4/e, p 541. Gilman, 8/e, p 1559.)* Pregnant women should not take more than a 25 percent increase in the normal dietary intake of vitamin A for it is definitely teratogenic, especially in the first trimester of pregnancy. Great caution is to be taken in premenopausal females in the therapy of acne and skin wrinkling in which tretinoin or isotretinoin is the therapeutic agent. None of the other vitamins is particularly teratogenic except perhaps vitamin D.

410. The answer is C. *(DiPalma, 4/e, pp 542, 546, 548. Gilman, 8/e, p 1524.)* Fat-soluble vitamins, especially vitamins A and D, can be stored in massive amounts and hence have a potential for serious toxicities. Water-soluble vitamins are easily excreted by the kidney and toxic accumulation rarely occurs.

411. The answer is A. *(DiPalma, 4/e, p 539. Gilman, 8/e, p 1524.)* The National Research Council has a Food and Nutrition Board, which has the function of selecting the levels of vitamins, minerals, and other substances necessary to achieve maximum nutritional health. The levels are reviewed periodically and determined by study of the nutritional needs of healthy persons. The Food and Drug Administration is responsible for labeling of nutritional products but does not determine the RDAs.

412. The answer is E. *(DiPalma, 4/e, p 748.)* The toxicity of isoniazid (INH) is mainly on the peripheral and central nervous systems. This is attributable to competition of INH with pyridoxal phosphate for apotryptophanase. This results in a relative deficiency of pyridoxine, which causes peripheral neuritis, insomnia, and muscle twitching among other effects.

413. The answer is C. *(DiPalma, 4/e, p 573. Gilman, 8/e, p 922.)* Dioctyl sodium sulfosuccinate (docusate) is a detergent that, when given orally, softens the stool and prevents straining. Mineral oil also softens the stool, but it tends to inhibit absorption of fat-soluble vitamins and other nutrients.

Castor oil, phenolphthalein, and cascara are strong laxatives and cause watery stools.

414. The answer is D. *(DiPalma, 4/e, pp 565–566. Gilman, 8/e, p 910.)* Sucralfate is a sulfated disaccharide that contains polyaluminum hydroxide. It has primarily protective properties and attaches firmly to ulcer craters. It has no significant acid-neutralizing properties.

415–416. The answers are 415-G, 416-I. *(DiPalma, 4/e, pp 539–556. Gilman, 8/e, pp 1523–1570.)* Phytonadione, the fat-soluble form of vitamin K, is often not included in so-called one-a-day vitamin preparations because it is so ubiquitous in the usual diet. Only in liver disease does a deficiency of the vitamin occur.

Calcitriol (1,25-D_3) is the most active form of vitamin D. It is formed by the kidney. When the calcium blood level rises, the kidney produces 24,25-D_3, a much less active form. Vitamin D can be manufactured in the body by the action of sunlight on the skin. Its main action is to increase calcium absorption in the gut. Thus, vitamin D subserves important hormonal functions in calcium homeostasis.

Levodopa is converted to dopamine in the peripheral tissues by dopa decarboxylase, which has as a cofactor pyridoxine. Excess of this vitamin will increase this reaction, which is an undesirable effect because dopamine does not cross the blood-brain barrier where the therapeutic effect is desired.

Menadione, the water-soluble form of vitamin K, should not be given to infants because of the high incidence of hemolysis and jaundice.

Alpha-tocopherol, or vitamin E, is relatively nontoxic and has antioxidant properties, e.g., preserving intracellular components such as ubiquinone.

417–418. The answers are 417-A, 418-C. *(DiPalma, 4/e, pp 539–556. Gilman, 8/e, pp 1523–1570.)* Angular stomatitis, dermatitis, and corneal vascularization are considered classic signs of human riboflavin deficiency, although multiple B vitamins may be involved.

Nicotinic acid (niacin) in doses of 1 to 3 g a day, over 100 times the RDA, causes a significant lowering of blood cholesterol. This is not an attribute of nicotinamide. Nicotinic acid and nicotinamide are both effective in curing pellagra. Large doses of nicotinic acid have been used in attempts to cure various psychoses, but this therapy is now discredited.

Vitamin C, which is sometimes recommended in large doses for the common cold and as a cure for cancer, is actually more useful as a method of acidifying urine and increasing the excretion of such abused drugs as phencyclidine.

Pyridoxine deficiency is most common in children on infant formulas that do not contain this vitamin. Deficiency of this vitamin causes convulsions.

The classic therapy of the bizarre CNS signs and symptoms of withdrawal in severe alcoholics (Wernicke's syndrome) is intravenous administration of thiamine plus glucose infusion. Alcoholics generally have other deficiencies of vitamins, especially riboflavin and niacin.

419–420. The answers are 419-C, 420-G. *(DiPalma, 4/e, pp 562–563, 570. Gilman, 8/e, pp 507–508, 902–904.)* Omeprazole, which is an inhibitor of the parietal cell H^+,K^+-ATPase pump, is the most effective means of decreasing gastric acidity. This makes it the ideal agent to treat Zollinger-Ellison syndrome, which results from increased gastric secretion due to gastrinomas.

Loperamide is an opiate that is poorly absorbed from the gastrointestinal tract but still retains the ability to inhibit peristalsis. It is useful in diarrheas that are just symptomatic and are not due to infection or organic pathology, such as inflammatory bowel disease.

421–422. The answers are 421-E, 422-C. *(DiPalma, 4/e, pp 572–574. Gilman, 8/e, pp 915–924.)* Lactulose is a disaccharide that is not absorbed and thus acts as an osmotic agent in the gut. In the colon, lactulose is broken down by bacteria to lactic, formic, and acetic acids plus carbon dioxide, which tend to also increase motility.

Phenolphthalein, like anthraquinones and other irritant phenolic compounds, is a stimulant laxative. Colonic peristalsis is increased by stimulation of sensory nerve endings in the mucosa of the intestine. Phenolphthalein also enhances entrance of water and salts into the bowel.

423–424. The answers are 423-F, 424-E. *(DiPalma, 4/e, pp 560–561. Gilman, 8/e, pp 898–911.)* Acetylcholine or vagal stimulation causes an increase in calcium in the parietal cell. This in turn stimulates protein kinase, which activates the H^+,K^+-ATPase pump to secrete H^+ ions and increase acidity. Blocking the action of acetylcholine with atropine-like drugs thus results in lower gastric acidity. Propantheline is an anticholinergic that has advantages over atropine and has been widely used to treat peptic ulcer.

Prostaglandins, especially E_2 and I_2, stimulate inhibitory G protein, which controls adenylate cyclase, so as to decrease the production of cyclic AMP and thus decrease the action of the H^+,K^+-ATPase pump through protein kinase. Aspirin and other NSAIDs inhibit the synthesis of prostaglandins, allowing stimulatory G protein to be activated by other mechanisms and thus allowing the parietal cell to secrete more acid. Misoprostol, a synthetic prostaglandin, is used to antagonize this action of aspirin and NSAIDs in patients who must take these drugs and who are at risk of developing peptic ulcers.

Endocrine System

Anabolic Steroids
- Dromostanolone propionate
- Methandrostenolone
- Nandrolone decanoate
- Nandrolone phenpropionate
- Oxandrolone
- Oxymetholone
- Stanozolol

Corticosteroids
- Beclomethasone
- Cortisone
- Dexamethasone
- Fludrocortisone
- Hydrocortisone
- Prednisone*
- Methylprednisolone
- Metyrapone
- Spironolactone
- Triamcinolone

Corticotropins
- Corticotropin (ACTH)*
- Cosyntropin

Female Sex Hormones and Oral Contraceptives
- Chlorotrianisene*
- Conjugated estrogens
- Danazol*
- Desogestrel
- Dienestrol
- Diethylstilbestrol
- Estradiol
- Estrone
- Estropipate
- Ethinyl estradiol
- Ethynodiol
- Hydroxyprogesterone
- Leuprolide*
- Levonorgestrel
- Luteinizing hormone-releasing hormone
- Medroxyprogesterone
- Megestrol
- Mestranol
- Mifepristone
- Norethindrone
- Norethynodrel
- Norgestrel
- Quinestrol
- Tamoxifen*

Fertility Agents
- Bromocriptine*
- Clomiphene*
- Human chorionic gonadotropin (hCG)
- Human menopausal gonadotropin (hMG)

Hyperglycemic Agents
- Diazoxide
- Glucagon*

Insulins
- Extended insulin zinc suspension
- Insulin injection
- Insulin zinc suspension
- Isophane (NPH)
- 70% Isophane insulin suspension + 30% insulin injection
- 50% Isophane insulin suspension + 50% insulin injection

Male Sex Hormones
- Finasteride

- Fluoxymesterone
- Flutamide
- Methyltestosterone*
- Nafarelin
- Testosterone*
- Testosterone cypionate
- Testosterone enanthate
- Testosterone propionate
- Spironolactone

Oral Hypoglycemic Agents
- Acetohexamide
- Chlorpropamide
- Glipizide
- Glyburide
- Tolazamide
- Tolbutamine*
- Metformin

Parathyroid Drugs
- Calcitonin*
- Calcitriol
- Calcifediol
- Dihydrotachysterol
- Ergocalciferol
- Etidronate*
- Gallium nitrate
- Parathyroid hormone (PTH)
- Pamidronate
- Phosphates
- Plicamycin (mithramycin)
- Vitamin D*

Thyroid Drugs
- Dessicated thyroid*
- Iodide (Lugol's solution)
- Levothyroxine
- Liothyronine
- Liotrix
- Methimazole
- Propylthiouracil*
- Protirelin
- Radioactive iodine (^{131}I)

DIRECTIONS: Each question below contains five suggested responses. Select the **one best** response to each question.

425. The mechanism of action of etidronate disodium (Didronel) is most likely related to

(A) an unusual form of phosphorus
(B) inhibition of both normal and abnormal bone resorption
(C) hyperphosphatemia
(D) excretion unchanged in the urine
(E) inhibition of formation of hydroxyapatite crystals

426. Glucocorticoid synthesis is under direct control of

(A) the hypothalamus
(B) the posterior pituitary
(C) the adrenal medulla
(D) corticotropin-releasing factor
(E) corticotropin (ACTH)

427. A substance that enhances the probability of ovulation by blocking the inhibitory effect of estrogens and thus stimulating the release of gonadotropin from the pituitary is

(A) oxymetholone (Anadrol-50)
(B) clomiphene (Clomid)
(C) diethylstilbestrol
(D) ethinyl estradiol
(E) progesterone

428. A naturally occurring substance useful in treating Paget's disease of bone is

(A) etidronate (Didronel)
(B) cortisol
(C) calcitonin (Calcimar)
(D) parathyroid hormone
(E) thyroxine

429. Isophane insulin suspension (NPH) differs from extended insulin zinc suspension (Ultralente) in which of the following actions?

(A) It activates receptor tyrosine kinases
(B) It causes movement of intracellular glucose transporters to the cell membrane
(C) Following subcutaneous injection, it reaches peak plasma concentrations by 6 to 10 h
(D) It has a longer duration of action
(E) It increases lipogenesis

430. The preferred thyroid preparation for maintenance replacement therapy is which of the following drugs?

(A) Desiccated thyroid
(B) Liothyronine (Cytomel)
(C) Protirelin (Thypinone)
(D) Levothyroxine (Levothroid)
(E) Liotrix (Euthroid)

431. A patient becomes markedly tetanic following a recent thyroidectomy. This symptom can be rapidly reversed by the administration of

(A) vitamin D
(B) calcitonin (Calcimar)
(C) parathyroid hormone
(D) plicamycin (mithramycin)
(E) calcium gluconate

432. As compared with finasteride (Proscar), flutamide (Eulexin)

(A) acts as an antiestrogen
(B) inhibits 5α-reductase
(C) can cause impotence
(D) blocks androgen receptors
(E) reduces levels of dihydrotestosterone

433. Metyrapone is useful in testing the endocrine functioning of the

(A) α cells of pancreatic islets
(B) β cells of pancreatic islets
(C) neurohypophysis
(D) pituitary-adrenal axis
(E) Leydig cells of testes

434. Of the following mechanisms of anti-inflammatory and immunosuppressive effects of glucocorticoids, which one is uniformly observed?

(A) Increased influx of leukocytes to the site of inflammation
(B) Reduced formation of lipocortins
(C) Reduced capillary permeability and edema at the inflammatory site
(D) Increased prostaglandin formation
(E) Enhanced formation of interleukins (IL-1, IL-2)

435. Bromocriptine (Parlodel) is used to treat some cases of amenorrhea because it

(A) stimulates release of gonadotropin-releasing hormone
(B) stimulates the ovary directly
(C) is an estrogen antagonist that enhances gonadotropin release
(D) inhibits prolactin release
(E) increases the synthesis of follicle-stimulating hormone

436. Tamoxifen (Nolvadex) is used to treat some breast cancers because of its ability to

(A) utilize its androgenic properties in retarding tumor growth
(B) prevent estrogen synthesis by the ovary
(C) enhance glucocorticoid treatment
(D) act as an estrogen antagonist
(E) act as a potent progestin

437. Which one of the following statements most accurately describes oxytocin?

(A) It is used for postpartum bleeding
(B) It is approved for use in elective induction of labor
(C) Overdosage can cause a sustained tetanic contraction
(D) It causes a large increase in blood pressure
(E) It inhibits milk ejection

438. The most dangerous adverse reaction to the administration of methimazole (Tapazole) is

(A) hypothyroidism
(B) arthralgia
(C) jaundice
(D) agranulocytosis
(E) renal toxicity

439. The initial and crucial event that enables tolbutamide (Orinase) to cause the pancreatic β cells to release insulin is

(A) increased potassium efflux
(B) binding to receptors on the ATP-sensitive K^+ channels
(C) closing of voltage-dependent calcium channels
(D) decreased phosphorylation reactions
(E) hyperpolarization

440. The treatment of myxedema coma can include which of the following agents?

(A) Thyroglobulin
(B) Levothyroxine
(C) Lithium
(D) Propylthiouracil
(E) Protirelin (Relefact TRH)

441. The "minipill" containing only a progestin, rather than a combination estrogen-progestin oral contraceptive, was developed because progestin alone

(A) results in less depression and cholestatic jaundice
(B) is a more effective contraceptive agent than the two combined
(C) results in a more regular menstrual cycle
(D) is thought to be less likely to induce endometriosis
(E) is thought to be less likely to induce cardiovascular disorders

442. Parathyroid hormone has which one of the following effects?

(A) Increased mobilization of calcium from bone
(B) Decreased active absorption of calcium from the small intestine
(C) Decreased renal tubular reabsorption of calcium
(D) Decreased resorption of phosphate from bone
(E) Decreased excretion of phosphate

DIRECTIONS: Each numbered question or incomplete statement below is NEGATIVELY phrased. Select the **one best** lettered response.

443. The general structure for thyroid hormones is shown below. In order for this structure to acquire significant hormone activity, all the following modifications must take place EXCEPT that

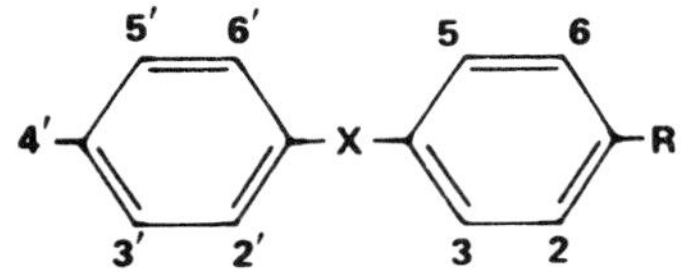

(A) the connection between the two aromatic rings should be by ether, thioether, or methylene linkage
(B) the R side chain on carbon 1 should be aliphatic and contain a carboxyl group
(C) halogenation or methylation is necessary at positions 3 and 5
(D) a hydroxyl group should be on position 3′
(E) position 4′ should have a hydroxyl group or a group capable of being metabolically converted to hydroxyl

444. Drugs that bind to receptors in the plasma membrane and enhance levels of cyclic 3′,5′-adenosine monophosphate (cAMP) include all the following EXCEPT

(A) adrenocorticotropic hormone (ACTH)
(B) calcitonin (Calcimar)
(C) isoproterenol (Isuprel)
(D) hydrocortisone
(E) glucagon

445. True statements about testosterone include all the following EXCEPT

(A) it is biotransformed primarily in the liver
(B) it enhances the excretion of sodium and water
(C) it has a stimulatory effect on hematopoietic cells
(D) it attaches to a receptor on the X chromosome
(E) it is converted to an active metabolite, dihydrotestosterone (DHT)

446. True statements concerning triiodothyronine (T_3) or thyroxine (T_4) include all the following EXCEPT

(A) T_3 readily penetrates cellular membrane
(B) T_3 attaches to cytoplasmic binders
(C) halogenase converts T_4 to T_3
(D) T_3 binds to receptors in the nucleus
(E) T_4 is actively transported into the cell

447. Inhibition of the peripheral conversion of T_4 to T_3 by the liver and kidney is caused by all the following drugs EXCEPT

(A) propranolol (Inderal)
(B) amiodarone (Cordarone)
(C) hydrocortisone
(D) methimazole (Tapazole)
(E) propylthiouracil (PTU)

448. All the following are steroid compounds EXCEPT

(A) mestranol
(B) clomiphene (Clomid)
(C) ethynodiol diacetate (Demulen)
(D) norethindrone (Norlutin)
(E) beclomethasone

449. True statements about dexamethasone (Decadron) include all the following EXCEPT

(A) it can stimulate lung maturation in the fetus
(B) it is used for the diagnosis of Cushing's syndrome
(C) it has minimal mineralocorticoid activity
(D) it is a short-acting glucocorticoid
(E) it is potentially ulcerogenic

450. Abuse of anabolic steroids by athletes can result in all the following EXCEPT

(A) retention of fluid
(B) feminization in males
(C) decreased spermatogenesis
(D) depression
(E) anorexia

451. Drugs that increase the need for insulin include all the following EXCEPT

(A) epinephrine
(B) hydrocortisone
(C) chlorthalidone (Hygroton)
(D) dexamethasone (Decadron)
(E) ethanol (acute ingestion)

452. Drugs that enter the cytoplasm of a cell and then bind to a specific receptor include all the following EXCEPT

(A) trihexyphenidyl (Artane)
(B) triamcinolone (Aristocort)
(C) mestranol
(D) fludrocortisone (Florinef)
(E) calcitriol (Rocaltrol)

453. Accurate statements about calcitriol (Rocaltrol) include all the following EXCEPT

(A) it is formed in the kidney from calcifediol by hydroxylation
(B) it may cause arrhythmias in digitalized patients
(C) it has a rapid onset of action
(D) it is 25-OH_3-vitamin D_3
(E) it enhances intestinal absorption of calcium

454. Adverse reactions to norethindrone include all the following EXCEPT

(A) acne
(B) weight gain
(C) hirsutism
(D) cholestatic jaundice
(E) venous thromboembolic disease

455. Adverse reactions to administration of chlorpropamide (Diabinese) include all the following EXCEPT

(A) water retention
(B) increased tolerance to ethanol
(C) hypoglycemia
(D) hyponatremia
(E) exacerbation of peptic ulcers

456. True statements about danazol (Danocrine) include all the following EXCEPT

(A) it is a testosterone derivative
(B) it can cause edema
(C) it can cause gynecomastia
(D) it can decrease HDL cholesterol
(E) it is indicated in endometriosis

457. Hypervitaminosis D produces all the following effects EXCEPT

(A) nephrocalcinosis
(B) polyuria
(C) osteoporosis
(D) polydipsia
(E) mild alkalosis

458. Adverse reactions associated with methylprednisolone include all the following EXCEPT

(A) osteoporosis
(B) peptic ulceration
(C) increased susceptibility to infection
(D) hypoglycemia
(E) edema

459. Glyburide (Micronase) has all the following attributes EXCEPT

(A) it is mildly diuretic
(B) it promotes the release of insulin
(C) it is a second-generation oral hypoglycemic agent
(D) its duration of action is 12 to 24 h and the drug may be given once a day
(E) it may decrease tolerance to ethanol

460. All the following drugs can cause hyperglycemia and hypokalemia EXCEPT

(A) hydrocortisone
(B) chlorpropamide (Diabinese)
(C) hydrochlorothiazide
(D) bumetanide (Bumex)
(E) prednisone

461. Spironolactone (Aldactone) is a useful diuretic with all the following effects EXCEPT

(A) it acts as a competitive antagonist
(B) it is used to treat hirsutism in women
(C) it is indicated in primary hyperaldosteronism
(D) it may cause hypokalemia
(E) it may cause gynecomastia

462. All the following compounds reduce the effectiveness of chlorpropamide EXCEPT

(A) phenobarbital
(B) chlorothiazide
(C) furosemide
(D) diazoxide
(E) salicylates

DIRECTIONS: Each group of questions below consists of lettered headings followed by a set of numbered items. For each numbered item select the **one** lettered heading with which it is **most** closely associated. Each lettered heading may be used **once, more than once, or not at all.**

Questions 463–465

Match each clinical use or entity below with the most appropriate drug.

(A) Mifepristone
(B) Spironolactone (Aldactone)
(C) Aminoglutethimide (Cytadren)
(D) Leuprolide
(E) Fludrocortisone (Florinef)

463. An abortifacient

464. Mineralocorticoid replacement therapy in primary adrenal insufficiency

465. Advanced prostate cancer

Questions 466–468

For each inhibitory effect on the synthesis of thyroid hormone listed below, select the agent that causes it.

(A) Sodium thiocyanate
(B) Methimazole (Tapazole)
(C) Triiodothyronine
(D) Radioactive iodine
(E) Iodide

466. Inhibits, by acting as a competitor, the accumulation of iodide in thyroid follicular cells

467. Inhibits the peroxidase-catalyzed oxidation of iodide and thus interferes with the incorporation of iodide into an organic structure

468. Inhibits the peroxidase-catalyzed coupling of iodotyrosines to form iodothyronines

Questions 469–471

Match each statement with the appropriate drug.

(A) Spironolactone (Aldactone)
(B) Furosemide (Lasix)
(C) Clomiphene (Clomid)
(D) Propranolol (Inderal)
(E) Medroxyprogesterone acetate
(F) Chlorpropamide (Diabinese)
(G) Plicamycin (Mithracin)
(H) Phentolamine (Regitine)
(I) Liothyronine (Cytomel)
(J) Calcitriol
(K) Fluoxymesterone (Halotestin)
(L) Nafarelin (Synarel)

469. An agent that is often useful in temporarily blocking the peripheral manifestations of hyperthyroidism

470. A cytotoxic antibiotic used to treat hypercalcemia associated with malignancies

471. An agent that produces changes in the cervical mucus and endometrium and suppresses ovulation

Questions 472–474

Match each statement with the correct drug.

(A) Aldosterone
(B) Clomiphene (Clomid)
(C) Diazoxide (Proglycem)
(D) Fludrocortisone (Florinef)
(E) Isophane insulin
(F) Methimazole (Tapazole)
(G) Ethinyl estradiol
(H) Norethindrone
(I) Norethynodrel
(J) Propylthiouracil
(K) Salicylates
(L) Spironolactone (Aldactone)
(M) Tamoxifen (Nolvadex)
(N) Triamcinolone (Aristocort)

472. This drug promotes the synthesis of factors II, VII, IX, and X and may interfere with the effect of warfarin or may result in thromboembolic phenomena

473. The therapeutic effect of this drug is reduced by glucocorticoids, dextrothyroxine, epinephrine, hydrochlorothiazide, and levothyroxine

474. This drug reduces the growth of facial hair in idiopathic hirsutism or hirsutism secondary to androgen excess

Endocrine System
Answers

425. The answer is E. *(DiPalma, 4/e, pp 594–595. Gilman, 8/e, pp 1509–1510.)* Etidronate is used in the treatment of Paget's disease of bone. The compound is classified as a diphosphonate. It can be administered orally or by injection. The drug affects both normal and abnormal bone resorption and appears to reduce the activity of osteoclasts and osteoblasts. It inhibits the formation, growth, and dissolution of hydroxyapatite crystals, which is probably its main mechanism of action. There occurs a significant reduction in serum calcium following several days of intravenous therapy with etidronate. The drug has a half-life of about 6 h and is excreted unchanged in the urine. Etidronate has also been used to treat patients with hypercalcemia that may be associated with various neoplastic diseases.

426. The answer is E. *(DiPalma, 4/e, pp 638–639. Gilman, 8/e, pp 1432–1436.)* Glucocorticoid synthesis is under the control of corticotropin (adrenocorticotropic hormone, ACTH). In response to the release of corticotropin-releasing factor (CRF), corticotropin is elaborated from the anterior pituitary gland. It is a polypeptide of 39 amino acids. In the body, cortisol (hydrocortisone) exerts a negative feedback mechanism to suppress the release of corticotropin. Corticotropin affects lipid metabolism by producing a stimulatory effect on lipolysis, which results in an elevated plasma concentration of free fatty acids. The drug is used in the diagnosis of adrenal insufficiency (e.g., primary adrenal insufficiency). When it is given intravenously, its half-life is short, lasting about 15 min. A synthetic form of corticotropin is cosyntropin, which contains only the first 24 amino acids of the peptide.

427. The answer is B. *(DiPalma, 4/e, pp 619–620. Gilman, 8/e, pp 1395–1396.)* Clomiphene (Clomid) is an effective fertility drug that can lead to multiple pregnancies. Clomiphene has been termed an antiestrogen because its stimulant effect on the secretion of pituitary gonadotropins is thought to be the consequence of its blocking the inhibitory effect of estrogens on gonadotropin secretion. Side effects of this drug can include alopecia, breast engorgement, and hot flashes. Oxymetholone is an orally effective anabolic steroid.

428. The answer is C. *(DiPalma, 4/e, pp 591–595. Gilman, 8/e, pp 1507–1510.)* Calcitonin is useful in the therapy of Paget's disease of bone (osteitis deformans). Calcitonin therapy reduces urinary hydroxyproline excretion and serum alkaline phosphatase activity and provides some symptomatic relief. Presumably these effects result from the ability of calcitonin to inhibit bone resorption. Side effects of long-term therapy with this hormone can include nausea, edema of the hands, and urticaria. The appearance of neutralizing antibodies may explain the development of resistance to treatment. Etidronate is a synthetic drug that is useful in Paget's disease. The compound is orally effective and lacks the antigenicity associated with calcitonin.

429. The answer is D. *(DiPalma, 4/e, pp 37–39, 599–602. Gilman, 8/e, pp 1469–1470, 1476–1477.)* Isophane insulin suspension (NPH) is obtained from animal sources (beef and pork) and by recombinant DNA techniques to yield human insulin. Protamine and zinc are contained in NPH insulin (neutral protamine Hagedorn). Following subcutaneous injection it has a maximum effect of 8 to 10 h that corresponds to its peak plasma concentrations (6 to 10 h). The duration of action is 18 to 26 h, which is shorter than the duration of action of extended insulin zinc suspension (Ultralente). On the cellular membrane, insulin binds to receptor tyrosine kinases. The activation of these receptor tyrosine kinases leads to phosphorylation reactions and the movement of glucose transporters from the intracellular space to the membranes, where they facilitate the entrance of glucose into the cell. Insulin lowers plasma glucose levels, increases lipogenesis, decreases lipolysis and ketogenesis, and enhances the uptake of amino acids to promote protein synthesis and growth of tissues.

430. The answer is D. *(AMA Drug Evaluations Annual, 1993, pp 991–993. DiPalma, 4/e, pp 587–589.)* The drug of choice for maintenance replacement therapy of hypothyroidism is levothyroxine (T_4). Monitoring of plasma blood levels of T_3 and T_4 from the administration of levothyroxine causes less difficulty than the monitoring of plasma hormone levels from liothyronine (T_3), since considerable fluctuation can occur with plasma concentrations of T_3. In addition T_3 has a shorter half-life. Liotrix is a mixture of T_4 and T_3 in a ratio of 4 : 1 that is designed to resemble the physiologic secretion of the thyroid gland. When liotrix is administered, the T_4 component is converted to T_3 in the body, and T_3, therefore, is actually not needed. It does not appear that liotrix provides any therapeutic advantage over levothyroxine by itself for the usual treatment of hypothyroidism. The treatment of hypothyroidism with desiccated thyroid is obsolete. Protirelin, a synthetic tripeptide, is chemically identical to thyrotropin-releasing hormone (TRH). This compound is used for the diagnosis of mild cases of hypothyroidism or hyperthyroidism.

431. The answer is E. *(DiPalma, 4/e, pp 591–594. Gilman, 8/e, pp 1247, 1507–1517.)* Administration of intravenous calcium gluconate would immediately correct the tetany that might occur in a patient in whom a thyroidectomy was recently performed. Parathyroid hormone would act more slowly but could be given for its future stabilizing effect. Long-term control of a patient after a thyroidectomy can be obtained with vitamin D and dietary therapy. Calcitonin is a hypocalcemic antagonist of parathyroid hormone. Plicamycin (mithramycin) is used to treat Paget's disease and hypercalcemia. The dose employed is about one-tenth the amount used for plicamycin's cytotoxic action.

432. The answer is D. *(DiPalma, 4/e, pp 636–637. Gilman, 8/e, p 1428.)* Finasteride is classified as an inhibitor of androgen synthesis and is used in the treatment of benign prostatic hyperplasia. Continuous administration of the drug increases urinary flow and relieves symptoms of urinary obstruction by decreasing the size of the enlarged prostate. The compound is not effective in all cases of benign prostatic hypertrophy. Finasteride prevents the conversion of testosterone to dihydrotestosterone (DHT) by inhibiting the enzyme 5α-reductase. Since the size of the prostate gland depends on DHT, as the levels of DHT are decreased, the hypertrophy of the gland is reduced. The drug is given orally on a continuous basis. There is extensive biotransformation of drug with excretion of the metabolites in the urine and feces. Reported side effects of finasteride include impotence and decreased libido. An example of a drug that is a competitive inhibitor of the androgen receptor is flutamide, which is indicated in the treatment of metastatic prostatic carcinoma.

433. The answer is D. *(DiPalma, 4/e, p 647. Gilman, 8/e, p 1458.)* Metyrapone (Metopirone), because it decreases serum levels of cortisol by inhibiting the 11β-hydroxylation of steroids in the adrenal, can be used to assess the function of the pituitary-adrenal axis. When metyrapone is administered orally or intravenously to normal persons, the adenohypophysis will secrete an increased amount of adrenocorticotropic hormone (ACTH). This will cause a normal adrenal gland to synthesize increased amounts of 17-hydroxylated steroids that can be measured in the urine. However, patients who have disease of the hypothalamico-pituitary complex are not able to respond to administration of metyrapone by producing increased amounts of ACTH; consequently, no increased levels of 17-hydroxylated steroids would be detected in the urine. Before administering the drug, the ability of the adrenal gland to respond to ACTH must be tested.

434. The answer is C. *(DiPalma, 4/e, pp 640–643. Gilman, 8/e, pp 1442–1445.)* Glucocorticoid compounds are used in therapy because of their anti-inflammatory and immunosuppressive properties. These steroids prevent the movement of neutrophils from the blood to the site of inflammation and cause a redistribution of leukocytes, which also reduces their influx to the site of inflammation. Glucocorticoids decrease the synthesis of prostaglandins by causing the production of lipocortin, which inhibits the enzyme phospholipase A_2. With the inhibition of phospholipase A_2, arachidonic acid is not released and as a consequence the synthesis of the prostaglandins is decreased or prevented. Glucocorticoids decrease capillary permeability and edema in the site of inflammation by decreasing vasodilation. These drugs inhibit the effects of interleukin 1 (IL-1), interleukin 2 (IL-2), tumor necrosis factor (TNF), macrophage migration inhibitory factor (MIF), and other components of the inflammatory and immune responses.

435. The answer is D. *(DiPalma, 4/e, p 628. Gilman, 8/e, p 1346.)* High prolactin levels in the serum result in amenorrhea, for reasons that are not known. Bromocriptine inhibits prolactin secretion through its dopaminergic action. This compound, a semisynthetic ergot derivative, appears to be a dopamine receptor agonist. It is administered orally to the patient, and in most cases menses occurs after a month of therapy.

436. The answer is D. *(DiPalma, 4/e, p 619. Gilman, 8/e, pp 1207, 1256–1257.)* Tamoxifen is an estrogen antagonist used in the treatment of breast cancer. Postmenopausal women with metastases to soft tissue and whose tumors contain an estrogen receptor are more likely to respond to this agent. Little benefit is derived from tamoxifen if the tumor does not have estrogen receptors.

437. The answer is C. *(Gilman, 8/e, pp 935–937, 948. Katzung, 6/e, pp 573–574.)* Oxytocin is used to induce or stimulate medically indicated labor; it should not be used for elective inductions. When used for inductions, it should be administered intravenously so that the rate of infusion can be controlled. If too much oxytocin is administered, a sustained tetanic contraction can result, which may rupture the uterus or cause fetal hypoxia. Oxytocin can cause milk ejection.

438. The answer is D. *(DiPalma, 4/e, p 588. Gilman, 8/e, pp 1373–1376.)* Methimazole is classified as a thioamide and is used in the treatment of hyperthyroidism. It prevents the organification of iodide by blocking the oxidation of iodide to active iodine and also inhibits coupling of iodotyrosines. Excessive treatment with this drug may induce hypothyroidism. Some other adverse reactions reported for methimazole include skin rash, fever, jaundice, nephritis, arthralgia, and edema. Agranulocytosis, which is a very serious reaction and may be fatal, is the most dangerous adverse reaction, but it occurs in less than 1 percent of patients. Patients should be carefully monitored while they are taking this medication because agranulocytosis appears without warning.

439. The answer is B. *(DiPalma, 4/e, pp 598–599. Gilman, 8/e, pp 1484–1485.)* Tolbutamide is an oral hypoglycemic agent that is classified as a sulfonylurea derivative. This compound is used in the treatment of non-insulin-dependent diabetes mellitus (NIDDM, or type II). For hypoglycemic action, tolbutamide needs functional β cells in the pancreas, since it is ineffective in depancreatized or severely insulin-deficient patients. Sulfonylurea compounds stimulate the release of insulin from the pancreas by a proposed mechanism of action involving the initial binding of the drug to a receptor on the ATP-sensitive potassium channels in the cell. As a consequence of this drug-receptor interaction, there is an inhibition of potassium efflux from the cell, which then produces depolarization of the membrane. The depolarization of the membrane opens voltage-dependent calcium channels to allow the entrance of calcium into the cell. The increased calcium concentration stimulates phosphorylation reactions, followed by the process of exocytosis, which causes the release of insulin from the *β* cells. Other drugs, such as diazoxide and epinephrine, reduce insulin secretion by causing hyperpolarization of the cell, decreasing calcium ion influx, and thereby preventing the process of exocytosis for the release of insulin.

440. The answer is B. *(AMA Drug Evaluations Annual, 1993, p 988. DiPalma, 4/e, pp 587–589.)* Myxedema coma is a medical emergency and should be treated as soon as the diagnosis is established. Treatment involves the use of several drugs to correct this condition. It appears that the selection of either levothyroxine, liothyronine, or liotrix is appropriate. Levothyroxine, however, is the drug of choice. Supportive treatment of symptoms is also indicated. Maintenance of respiration and administration of fluids and electrolytes, along with glucose if hypoglycemia is diagnosed, should be provided. Since adrenal insufficiency may be present, administration of glucocorticoids is initially recommended. Thyroglobulin, a protein of high molecular weight, is a component of the thyroid gland. Although preparations are available, this drug is not indicated in myxedema coma. Protirelin is a synthetic thyrotropin-stimulating hormone used in the diagnosis of thyroid function. Although lithium was once tested as a drug to treat hyperthyroidism because it induced hypothyroidism, lithium has no place in the therapy of hyperthyroidism. In addition, propylthiouracil is an antithyroid drug used in the management of hyperthyroidism.

441. The answer is E. *(DiPalma, 4/e, pp 621–627. Gilman, 8/e, pp 1403–1407.)* The combination of estrogen and progestin is a more effective means of contraception than is progestin alone. Menstruation will occur with progestin alone, but it may be irregular. Estrogen is thought to cause the increased incidence of thrombophlebitis and cerebral and coronary thrombosis that is found in women taking combined oral contraceptives.

442. The answer is A. *(DiPalma, 4/e, pp 590–594. Gilman, 8/e, pp 1503–1507.)* Parathyroid hormone (PTH) is synthesized by and released from the parathyroid gland; increased synthesis of PTH is a response to low serum calcium concentrations. Resorption and mobilization of calcium and phosphate from bone are increased in response to elevated PTH concentrations. Replacement of body stores of calcium is enhanced by the capacity of PTH to promote increased absorption of calcium by the small intestine in concert with vitamin D, which is the primary factor that enhances intestinal calcium absorption. PTH also causes an increased renal tubular reabsorption of calcium and excretion of phosphate. As a consequence of these effects, the extracellular calcium concentration becomes elevated.

443. The answer is D. *(DiPalma, 4/e, pp 583–584. Gilman, 8/e, pp 1361–1365.)* According to extensive research on the relationship between structure and activity of thyronine derivatives, significant thyroid hormone activity would be characteristic of the structure below.

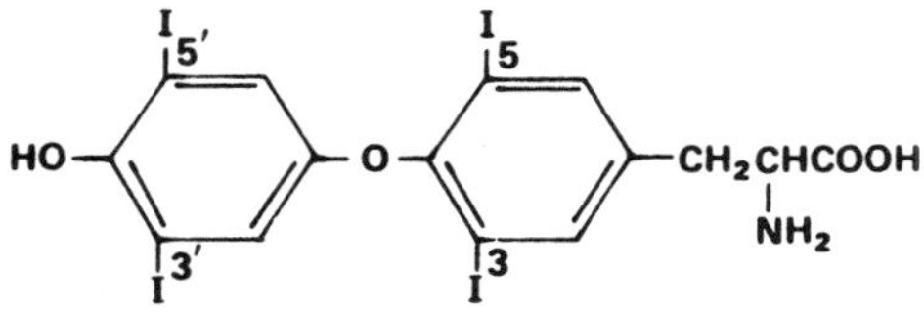

This structure is thyroxine, in which the R side chain is L-alanine, the aromatic rings are connected by an ether linkage, halogenation by iodine occurs on positions 3,5 and 3′,5′, and a hydroxyl group is attached to carbon 4′. Activity can be increased fourfold upon removing iodine from the 5′ position because 3′-monosubstituted compounds have more activity than 3′,5′-disubstituted derivatives of thyronine.

444. The answer is D. *(DiPalma, 4/e, pp 34–37, 640. Gilman, 8/e, pp 1437–1438.)* Cyclic AMP is an intracellular second messenger that is involved in the mechanism of action associated with adrenocorticotropic hormone, calcitonin, isoproterenol, and glucagon. These agents complex with a plasma membrane receptor that brings about the binding of guanosine triphosphate (GTP) to the coupling protein and the activation of adenylate cyclase. Adenylate cyclase catalyzes the formation of cAMP from ATP. In the cytoplasm cAMP activates cAMP-dependent protein kinase, which participates in the phosphorylation of specific substrate proteins (e.g., enzymes). The phosphorylated protein eventually induces the particular response on the target cell that is associated with the administered drug. The cellular mechanism of action of hydrocortisone, a glucocorticoid, is also related to proteins but not by the enhancement of cAMP production. Hydrocortisone is transported by simple diffusion across the membrane of the cell into the cytoplasm and binds to a specific receptor. The steroid-receptor complex is activated and enters the nucleus, where it regulates transcription of specific gene sequences into RNA. Eventually mRNA is translated to form specific proteins in the cytoplasm that are involved in the steroid-induced cellular response.

445. The answer is B. *(DiPalma, 4/e, pp 630–632, 634. Gilman, 8/e, pp 1418–1424.)* In many tissues testosterone is transformed into dihydrotestosterone (DHT) by 5α-reductase. This active metabolite is more potent than testosterone and appears to be responsible for the androgenic effects in the body. The affinity of dihydrotestosterone is 10 times that of testosterone for the androgen-receptor gene that is located on the X chromosome. The compound testosterone is eliminated from the body through biotransformation in the liver and excretion of its metabolites, 17-ketosteroids, in the urine. Adverse reactions of testosterone and its various derivatives include virilism in prepubertal males and masculinization in females. Some other untoward effects are liver dysfunction, hypercalcemia, and retention of sodium and water. Therapeutic uses of androgenic compounds are in the area of male hypogonadism, certain types of breast carcinomas, and anemia. Androgens are used in some forms of anemia because they cause the release of erythropoietin-stimulating factor, which increases production of red blood cells.

446. The answer is E. *(DiPalma, 4/e, pp 585–586. Katzung, 6/e, pp 581–582.)* The receptors that bind the physiologic ligand of thyroid hormone appear to be located in the nucleus of the cell as opposed to the cytoplasmic location of steroid receptors. Both thyroxine (T_4) and triiodothyronine (T_3) enter the cell in the same manner, which is probably by passive diffusion. In the cytoplasm halogenase converts T_4 to T_3. T_3 can attach to cytoplasmic binders or enter the nucleus and bind to receptors. The T_3-receptor complex in association with DNA eventually directs the synthesis of new protein, which changes cellular activity to reflect the presence of thyroid hormone.

447. The answer is D. *(AMA Drug Evaluations Annual, 1993, pp 983–984, 992–993. DiPalma, 4/e, pp 583–587.)* Triiodothyronine (T_3) and thyroxine (T_4) are released from the thyroid gland and enter the circulation. T_4 is converted to T_3, which is more potent in activity, by the liver and kidney. This conversion reaction is inhibited by propranolol, amiodarone, hydrocortisone, and propylthiouracil. Although methimazole and propylthiouracil inhibit the enzymatic oxidation of iodide ion to active iodine, which is their principal mechanism as antithyroid drugs, only propylthiouracil can block the peripheral conversion of T_4 to T_3. Propranolol and hydrocortisone are used in the treatment of certain cases of hyperthyroidism, and whether the reduction in the conversion of T_4 to T_3 plays a significant role in their mechanism of action is not fully known. The compound amiodarone is an antiarrhythmic drug that is similar in chemical structure to thyroxine.

448. The answer is B. *(DiPalma, 4/e, pp 615, 619–620. Gilman, 8/e, pp 1395–1397.)* All the compounds listed in the question are steroids with the exception of clomiphene (Clomid), an estrogen analogue that lacks the essential feature of a steroid: a hydrogenated cyclopentenophenanthrene-ring system. Clomid is a derivative of the weakly estrogenic compound chlorotrianisene. The compound has high antiestrogenic activity that inhibits estrogenic feedback repression of gonadotropic secretion. Clomid is an effective fertility-inducing drug.

449. The answer is D. *(DiPalma, 4/e, pp 643–648. Katzung, 6/e, pp 595–600.)* The compound dexamethasone is classified as a long-acting ($t_{1/2}$ = 36 h) synthetic glucocorticoid. This drug is a 9α-fluoro, 16α-methyl derivative that possesses little or no mineralocorticoid activity. When dexamethasone is compared with hydrocortisone for mineralocorticoid potency at an equivalent dose, dexamethasone is rated as zero, while hydrocortisone is given a value of 1. It is reported that dexamethasone induces ulceration of the gastrointestinal tract. Glucocorticoids appear to stimulate production of acid and pepsin in the stomach. Dexamethasone is used to reduce the occurrence of respiratory distress syndrome in premature infants. This steroid stimulates lung maturation when large doses are given to the mother prior to early delivery. Dexamethasone is also used for diagnostic purposes. The drug is used in the diagnosis of Cushing's syndrome and has been employed in the differential diagnosis of depressive psychiatric states.

450. The answer is E. *(DiPalma, 4/e, p 635. Gilman, 8/e, pp 1425–1426.)* The use of anabolic steroids by athletes has become quite alarming in recent years. These steroids, which have androgenic and anabolic effects, are used to improve the performance of athletes in various competitive sports. Continued use of anabolic steroids induces mood changes as well as mental disorders from depression to psychosis. The androgenic properties of these drugs cause masculinization in females and may produce feminization in males. This latter effect is due to increased formation of estrogens. In addition, these steroids decrease production of endogenous testosterone by the testes and may cause a reduction in spermatogenesis. The weight gain that occurs with the administration of anabolic steroids may be due to fluid retention and an improved appetite rather than actual tissue growth. These drugs cause liver damage and increase the risk of cardiovascular diseases.

451. The answer is E. *(DiPalma, 4/e, pp 257, 457–460, 644.)* The regulation of levels of blood glucose by insulin and the general effectiveness of insulin are altered with the coadministration of other drugs. Epinephrine enhances glycogenolysis and thereby elevates glucose in the plasma. Glucocorticoids (e.g., hydrocortisone and dexamethasone) stimulate gluconeogenesis, reduce the peripheral utilization of glucose, and decrease the sensitivity of tissues to insulin. Chlorthalidone, a thiazide-related diuretic, may induce hyperglycemia by inhibition of the release of insulin and decrease use of glucose by peripheral tissues. In the presence of ethanol, the effect of insulin is enhanced. When ethanol is acutely ingested in sufficient quantities, the drug causes an alteration in carbohydrate metabolism that results in hypoglycemia. The exact mechanism of the hypoglycemic effect of ethanol is not known.

452. The answer is A. *(DiPalma, 4/e, pp 39–40, 316, 616, 630, 640.)* A variety of drugs that resemble steroid hormones in their structure can traverse cellular membranes and bind to specific cytoplasmic receptors. Triamcinolone (a glucocorticoid), fludrocortisone (a mineralocorticoid), mestranol (a sex steroid), and calcitriol (a vitamin D metabolite) all bind reversibly to the cytoplasmic receptor, which then undergoes an irreversible activation step. Next, the steroid-receptor complex enters the nucleus of the cell and regulates transcription of specific genes into RNA. Eventually mRNA is formed and causes the synthesis of specific proteins that mediate the steroid response. The response occurs 30 min to several hours following administration of the drug, since a period of time is required for formation of new proteins in the cell. Trihexyphenidyl is a synthetic anticholinergic drug that binds to muscarinic receptors associated with the cell membrane. This drug is used in the treatment of parkinsonism.

453. The answer is D. *(AMA Drug Evaluations Annual, 1993, p 2204. DiPalma, 4/e, pp 592–594.)* Vitamin D_3 is hydroxylated to 25-OHD_3 (calcifediol). Calcifediol is then hydroxylated in the kidney to the most active form of vitamin D, which is 1,25-$(OH)_2D_3$ (calcitriol). Calcitriol has a rapid onset of action and a short half-life. The administration of calcitriol causes the elevation of serum calcium levels by enhancing the intestinal absorption of calcium. Calcitriol is indicated in vitamin D deficiency, particularly in patients with chronic renal failure or renal tubular disease, hypoparathyroidism, osteomalacia, and rickets. In patients who are treated with a digitalis preparation, it is possible for a drug interaction to occur between digitalis and drugs, such as calcitriol, that can induce hypercalcemia. Elevation of serum calcium by calcitriol in the presence of digitalis glycosides can precipitate arrhythmias.

454. The answer is E. *(DiPalma, 4/e, pp 620–627. Katzung, 6/e, pp 615–624.)* Norethindrone is a 19-nortestosterone derivative. This progestational compound possesses a degree of androgenic and anabolic activity. The major use of norethindrone is as an oral contraceptive, alone or in combination with an estrogen. Some adverse reactions attributed to this progestational agent include increased appetite with weight gain, hirsutism, acne, seborrhea, and cholestatic jaundice. The risk of venous thromboembolic disease is associated with estrogenic agents.

455. The answer is B. *(AMA Drug Evaluations Annual, 1993, pp 1028–1032. DiPalma, 4/e, pp 604–608.)* The oral hypoglycemic agent chlorpropamide is a sulfonylurea compound. The drug is used to treat selected patients with non-insulin-dependent diabetes mellitus (NIDDM, type II). Chlorpropamide has a duration of action of 1 to 3 days. The adverse reaction of hypoglycemia appears to be more common with chlorpropamide than with the other sulfonylurea oral hypoglycemic agents. In addition, water retention and hyponatremia can be caused by chlorpropamide. This adverse reaction is due to an interaction between antidiuretic hormone (ADH) and chlorpropamide. In the collecting duct region of the nephron, chlorpropamide may enhance the effect of antidiuretic hormone and facilitate its release from the posterior pituitary gland. It is reported that chlorpropamide decreases the tolerance to ethanol—an interaction exhibited by flushing of the skin, particularly in the facial area. This disulfiram-like effect is attributed to the inhibition of the oxidation of acetaldehyde that is formed from the biotransformation of ethanol.

456. The answer is C. *(AMA Drug Evaluations Annual, 1993, pp 1076, 1091. DiPalma, 4/e, pp 620, 634.)* Danazol is a 17α-ethinyl testosterone derivative used to treat endometriosis. It appears to be more effective than an estrogen-progestin combination. Since danazol is an androgen derivative, some of the adverse reactions include liver dysfunction, virilism (acne, hirsutism, oily skin, reduced breast size), and reduction in high-density lipoprotein (HDL) cholesterol levels. Other adverse reactions reported for danazol are amenorrhea, weight gain, sweating, vasomotor flushing, and edema. When danazol therapy for endometriosis was compared with the estrogen-progestin regimen, few women discontinued the treatment with danazol because of adverse reactions.

457. The answer is E. *(DiPalma, 4/e, pp 592–594. Gilman, 8/e, pp 1514–1515.)* Enthusiastic overmedication with vitamin D may lead to a toxic syndrome called hypervitaminosis D. The initial symptoms can include weakness, nausea, weight loss, anemia, and mild acidosis. As the excessive doses are continued, signs of nephrotoxicity are manifested, such as polyuria, polydipsia, azotemia, and eventually nephrocalcinosis. In adults osteoporosis can occur. Also there is CNS impairment, which can result in mental retardation and convulsions.

458. The answer is D. *(DiPalma, 4/e, pp 644–648. Gilman, 8/e, pp 1446–1452.)* The incidence of adverse reactions with administration of methylprednisolone is related to dosage and duration. Psychoses, peptic ulceration with or without hemorrhage, increased susceptibility to infection, edema, osteoporosis, myopathy, and hypokalemic alkalosis can occur. Other adverse reactions include cataracts, hyperglycemia, arrest of growth in children, and iatrogenic Cushing's syndrome. The glucocorticoids are very effective drugs, but they can be very dangerous if not properly administered to a patient.

459. The answer is E. *(AMA Drug Evaluations Annual, 1993, pp 1028–1033. DiPalma, 4/e, pp 604–607.)* Glyburide is classified as a second-generation oral hypoglycemic agent. It causes hypoglycemia by stimulating the release of insulin from the pancreas and increases peripheral sensitivity to insulin. The drug is well absorbed upon oral administration and is biotransformed by the liver. Its duration of action is about 12 to 24 h, whereas the duration of action of chlorpropamide is 1 to 3 days. Glyburide has a mild course of action, whereas chlorpropamide can cause water retention and dilutional hyponatremia. In addition chlorpropamide may decrease tolerance to ethanol in that ethanol in the presence of chlorpropamide causes flushing of the skin, particularly in the facial area. Glyburide has not been reported to cause this effect when ethanol is consumed.

460. The answer is B. *(DiPalma, 4/e, pp 458–462, 606–607. Gilman, 8/e, pp 1438–1440, 1484–1485.)* The concurrent administration of hydrocortisone and an oral hypoglycemic agent, such as chlorpropamide, reduces the effectiveness of the hypoglycemic agent in controlling blood glucose levels in patients who have non-insulin-dependent diabetes mellitus. Hydrocortisone and prednisone induce hyperglycemia by enhancing gluconeogenesis in the liver and periphery. In addition the steroids also promote the release of glucagon from the cells of the pancreas to eventually increase blood glucose levels. Hydrocortisone possesses significant mineralocorticoid activity in addition to its glucocorticoid effect. The mineralocorticoid action of hydrocortisone alters electrolyte metabolism. Hydrocortisone enhances the retention of sodium and water in the body and augments the secretion of potassium, which can lead to hypokalemia. Prednisone also possesses a degree of mineralocorticoid activity and may produce hypokalemia. The diuretics hydrochlorothiazide and bumetanide can cause hypokalemia. In addition these diuretics cause hyperglycemia by inhibiting the release of insulin from the pancreas. If patients are to receive hydrocortisone and a loop or a thiazide diuretic, their potassium levels should be monitored to prevent potassium depletion.

461. The answer is D. *(DiPalma, 4/e, pp 463, 649. Katzung, 6/e, p 605.)* Spironolactone is an aldosterone antagonist. It and its active metabolite, canrenone, act as a competitive antagonist against aldosterone. The drug is used as a diuretic and in certain endocrine disorders. Spironolactone is indicated in primary hyperaldosteronism. In addition, it has been used to treat women with idiopathic hirsutism or hirsutism secondary to excessive androgens. This effect of spironolactone may be due to decreased androgen synthesis and an action in the hair follicle. As a diuretic agent spironolactone acts at the late distal tubule and collecting duct of the nephron to block the reabsorption of sodium and to promote conservation of potassium. The adverse reactions for spironolactone can include hyperkalemia, gastrointestinal effects, deepening of the voice, irregular menses, and gynecomastia.

462. The answer is E. *(DiPalma, 4/e, pp 586, 604, 607. Gilman, 8/e, pp 1482–1483.)* Oral hypoglycemic agents are used in the treatment of patients with non-insulin-dependent diabetes mellitus (NIDDM, or type II). Chlorpropamide is a sulfonylurea compound that regulates blood glucose levels by promoting the secretion of insulin from β cells in the pancreas. Caution must be exercised when other drugs are given concomitantly with oral hypoglycemic agents. The effectiveness of chlorpropamide can be reduced by drugs such as phenobarbital, rifampin, thiazide and loop diuretics, phenytoin, and diazoxide. Phenobarbital and rifampin induce the biotransformation of oral hypoglycemic agents. The thiazides (e.g., chlorothiazide) and loop diuretic drugs (e.g., furosemide) as well as diazoxide reduce the hypoglycemic effect of chlorpropamide by inhibiting the secretion of insulin from the pancreas. Examples of some drugs that enhance the hypoglycemic action of chlorpropamide and other such compounds are aspirin, ethanol, H_2-receptor antagonists, probenecid, and sulfonamides.

463–465. The answers are 463-A, 464-E, 465-D. *(AMA Drug Evaluations Annual, 1993, pp 969, 971, 977, 1153, 2040. DiPalma, 4/e, pp 463, 624, 636–637, 644–645, 649.)* Mifepristone is structurally related to norethindrone. This compound is classified as a progesterone antagonist with weak agonistic properties. It can induce an abortion by causing contraction of the myometrium, which leads to detachment of the embryo. The drug is used in a single or multiple dose followed by the administration of a prostaglandin to cause the abortion. Mifepristone is well absorbed following oral administration. It is biotransformed to several active products. Most of the parent compound and its metabolites are excreted in the feces. Presently, mifepristone is not available in the United States to be used as an abortifacient.

Fludrocortisone is a synthetic steroid compound that exhibits profound mineralocorticoid activity and some glucocorticoid activity. Electrolyte and water metabolisms are affected by the administration of this compound. Fludrocortisone promotes the reabsorption of sodium and the urinary excretion of potassium and hydrogen ions in the collecting duct of the nephron. The drug is indicated for mineralocorticoid replacement therapy in primary adrenal insufficiency.

Leuprolide is a peptide that is related to gonadotropin-releasing hormone or luteinizing hormone–releasing hormone. This agent is used to treat metastatic prostate carcinoma. A hypogonadal state is produced in the patient from the continuous administration of leuprolide. Testosterone levels in the body become significantly reduced.

466–468. The answers are 466-A, 467-B, 468-B. *(DiPalma, 4/e, pp 584, 587–589. Gilman, 8/e, pp 1363, 1371, 1373, 1377, 1379.)* Agents that can interfere directly or indirectly with the synthesis of thyroid hormone are called *thyroid inhibitors*. Thiocyanate, an ionic inhibitor, interferes with the ability of the thyroid to concentrate iodide by acting as a competitive inhibitor. Thiocyanate and other ionic inhibitors, such as perchlorate, nitrate, and fluoborate, are hydrated monovalent anions having a size similar to that of iodide.

Methimazole (Tapazole), together with propylthiouracil, is classified as an antithyroid drug that interferes directly with thyroid hormone synthesis. Antithyroid drugs interfere with the oxidation and incorporation of iodide into organic form and inhibit the formation of iodothyronines from the peroxidase-mediated coupling of iodotyrosines. These drugs may act by binding to peroxidase, by interacting with substrates, or by interfering with the production of hydrogen peroxide, which (in addition to oxygen) is a biologic oxidant required for the synthesis of thyroid hormones.

Iodide, most ancient of therapeutic agents for thyroid disorders, inhibits the secretion of thyroid hormone by retarding both the pinocytosis of colloid and proteolysis. This effect is observed in euthyroid as well as hyperthyroid persons.

Triiodothyronine is not classified as a thyroid inhibitor; it is an amino acid derivative of thyronine and results from the oxidative coupling of monoiodotyrosyl and diiodotyrosyl residues.

^{131}I, the most often used radioisotope of iodine, is rapidly absorbed by the thyroid and is deposited in follicular colloid. From the site of its deposition, ^{131}I causes fibrosis of the thyroid subsequent to pyknosis and necrosis of the follicular cells.

469–471. The answers are 469-D, 470-G, 471-E. *(DiPalma, 4/e, pp 134, 136, 589, 594, 623, 627. Gilman, 8/e, pp 1376, 1482.)* In patients who are suspected of having hyperthyroidism, propranolol may be administered to provide temporary relief of the peripheral manifestations of the disease while the patient is further evaluated. Propranolol suppresses adrenergic symptoms such as tremors and tachycardia. It has no effect on the release of thyroid hormones from the gland.

Plicamycin is an antineoplastic agent that belongs to the class of antibiotics. This drug may be used to treat hypercalcemia associated with malignancies. Its mechanism of action involves the inhibition of calcium reabsorption from bone. This effect leads to a reduction in serum calcium levels.

Medroxyprogesterone acetate is a progestin compound used as a contraceptive. It changes the cervical mucus and endometrium and suppresses ovulation. The drug is administered intramuscularly and is effective for 3 months. The prolonged effect of medroxyprogesterone acetate is probably related to its biotransformation. Adverse reactions that can occur include headache, weight gain, and depression.

472–474. The answers are 472-G, 473-E, 474-L. *(AMA Drug Evaluations Annual, 1993, pp 1030–1031, 1137. DiPalma, 4/e, pp 463–464, 617, 627.)* Ethinyl estradiol is a synthetic estrogen derivative that is orally effective. It is used in combination with progestins as an oral contraceptive. Ethinyl estradiol is also used alone in various gynecologic disorders such as menopausal symptoms, breast cancer in selected postmenopausal women, and prostatic carcinoma. A major adverse reaction with ethinyl estradiol and other estrogens involves the coagulation reaction. Estrogens increase the synthesis of vitamin K–dependent factors II, VII, IX, and X. The effect on the coagulation scheme can alter the prothrombin time of persons who are using oral anticoagulants (e.g., warfarin). In addition, estrogens can increase the incidence of thromboembolic disorders through their procoagulation effect.

In the therapy of diabetes mellitus the effectiveness of insulin to regulate glucose levels in the body can be reduced by simultaneous administration of other drugs. Glucose levels in the body are elevated by the administration of glucocorticoid (e.g., hydrocortisone), dextrothyroxine, epinephrine, thiazide diuretics (e.g., hydrochlorothiazide), and levothyroxine. The drug-induced hyperglycemia counteracts the hypoglycemic action of insulin preparations. In addition, any drug that induces hyperglycemia can also reduce the effectiveness of the oral hypoglycemic agents such as tolbutamide, acetohexamide, and glyburide.

Spironolactone is classified as a potassium-sparing diuretic. Spironolactone is a competitive inhibitor of aldosterone. It has a mild diuretic effect but is generally used with other diuretics such as thiazides or loop diuretics to prevent the development of hypokalemia. The drug is also used in endocrinology in the diagnosis and treatment of hyperaldosteronism. Another therapeutic use of spironolactone is in the treatment of hirsutism in females, whether it is idiopathic or related to excessive androgen secretion. The drug causes a decrease in the rate of growth and the density of facial hair, possibly through inhibition of excessive androgen production and an effect on the hair follicle.

Toxicology

- Air Pollutants
  - Benzene
  - Carbon monoxide
  - Carbon tetrachloride
  - Chloroform
  - Nitrogen dioxide
  - Ozone
  - Sulfur dioxide
  - Tetrachloroethylene
  - Toluene
  - 1,1,1-Trichloroethane
  - Trichloroethylene
- Alcohols
  - Ethanol
  - Methanol
  - Ethylene glycol
- Heavy Metals
  - Aluminum
  - Arsenic
  - Cadmium
  - Gold
  - Iron
  - Lead
  - Mercury
  - Zinc
- Heavy Metal Antagonists
  - Calcium disodium edetate
  - Deferoxamine
  - Dimercaprol
  - Penicillamine
- Herbicide
  - 2,4-Dichlorophenoxyacetic acid
- Organophosphorus Insecticides
  - Diazinon
  - Malathion
  - Parathion
  - Antidotes: atropine and pralidoxime
- Toxic Gas
  - Carbon monoxide
- Toxic Ion
  - Cyanide

DIRECTIONS: Each question below contains five suggested responses. Select the **one best** response to each question.

475. Convulsions caused by drug poisoning are most commonly associated with

(A) phenobarbital
(B) diazepam
(C) strychnine
(D) chlorpromazine
(E) phenytoin

476. Alkalinization of the urine with sodium bicarbonate is useful in the treatment of poisoning with

(A) aspirin (acetylsalicylic acid)
(B) amphetamine
(C) morphine
(D) phencyclidine
(E) cocaine

477. Which of the following is an agent useful in the treatment of severe poisoning by organophosphorus insecticides, such as parathion?

(A) Ethylenediaminetetraacetic acid (EDTA)
(B) Pralidoxime (2-PAM)
(C) *N*-Acetylcysteine
(D) Carbachol
(E) Diethyldithiocarbamic acid

478. *N*-Acetylbenzoquinoneimine is the hepatotoxic metabolite of which drug?

(A) Sulindac (Clinoril)
(B) Acetaminophen
(C) Isoniazid
(D) Indomethacin (Indocin)
(E) Procainamide

479. Rapid intravenous administration of this drug causes hypocalcemic tetany.

(A) Dimercaprol
(B) Edetate disodium
(C) Deferoxamine
(D) Penicillamine
(E) *N*-Acetylcysteine

480. Acute intermittent porphyria is a contraindication of the use of

(A) enflurane (Ethrane)
(B) nitrous oxide
(C) ketamine (Ketalar)
(D) diazepam (Valium)
(E) thiopental sodium

DIRECTIONS: Each numbered question or incomplete statement below is NEGATIVELY phrased. Select the **one best** lettered response.

481. All the following statements are valid mechanisms of drug interactions EXCEPT

(A) aspirin may increase the hypoprothrombinemic effect of dicumarol
(B) combining amphetamine and levothyroxine may cause cardiac tachyarrythmias
(C) amitriptyline may increase the sedative effect of ethanol
(D) cholestyramine enhances the hepatotoxicity of acetaminophen
(E) benztropine would increase the risk of urinary retention, paralytic ileus, and blurred vision associated with thioridazine

482. Characteristic features of arsenic poisoning include all the following EXCEPT

(A) acute poisoning causes severe diarrhea and difficulty swallowing
(B) signs of chronic poisoning include peripheral neuritis, hypotension, and anemia
(C) death following acute intoxication may be due to hypovolemic shock
(D) dimercaprol is the primary agent used in the treatment of chronic arsenic poisoning
(E) gingivitis, stomatitis, and salivation can occur

483. Cadmium poisoning is almost as common as lead and mercury poisoning. Its features include all the following EXCEPT

(A) it is commonly the main metal in certain types of batteries
(B) exposure to fumes causes dyspnea, substernal discomfort, myalgias, headaches, and vomiting
(C) chronic exposure results in severe liver injury
(D) the most common long-term toxicity is renal
(E) in Japan a cadmium intoxication syndrome is known as *itai-itai* (ouch-ouch) because of back, joint, and bone pain

484. Activated charcoal may be used to treat poisoning by all the following drugs EXCEPT

(A) phenobarbital
(B) carbamazepine (Tegretol)
(C) proxyphene (Darvon)
(D) lithium
(E) aspirin

485. Methanol is a frequent cause of poisoning in alcoholics. Methanol intoxication differs from ethanol intoxication in all the following ways EXCEPT

(A) blurred vision and hyperemia of the optic disc may develop
(B) it may produce bradycardia, coma, and seizures
(C) treatment includes administration of ethanol
(D) ascorbic acid corrects the metabolic alkalosis
(E) treatment may include hemodialysis

486. All the following drugs may produce a syndrome of flushing, headache, nausea, vomiting, sweating, hypotension, and confusion after ethanol consumption EXCEPT

(A) amitriptyline (Elavil)
(B) cefoperazine (Cefobid)
(C) acetohexamide (Dymelor)
(D) moxalactam (Moxane)
(E) disulfiram (Antabuse)

487. All the following statements are characteristic of carbon monoxide poisoning EXCEPT

(A) poisoning is effectively treated with 100% oxygen
(B) it binds to hemoglobin, reducing the oxygen-carrying capacity of blood
(C) carboxyhemoglobin levels below 15 percent rarely produce symptoms
(D) symptoms of poisoning include headache, convulsions, and respiratory and cardiovascular depression
(E) it inhibits ferricytochrome oxidase

488. Zinc is an essential element for normal growth and development. However, toxicity can occur from excessive exposure. Manifestations of chronic poisoning include all the following EXCEPT

(A) hyperamylasemia
(B) thrombocytopenia
(C) anemia
(D) encephalopathy
(E) fever

DIRECTIONS: Each group of questions below consists of lettered headings followed by a set of numbered items. For each numbered item select the **one** lettered heading with which it is **most** closely associated. Each lettered heading may be used **once, more than once, or not at all**.

Questions 489–490

Many drugs when given to a pregnant woman produce significant adverse effects on the fetus. For each of the drugs below, match the most likely adverse effect.

(A) Vaginal adenocarcinoma
(B) Congenital goiter, hypothyroidism
(C) Masculinization of female fetus
(D) Gray baby syndrome
(E) Prolonged neonatal hypoglycemia
(F) Kernicterus

489. Testosterone

490. Methimazole

Questions 491–492

For the agents below, select the specific antidote.

(A) Leucovorin
(B) Naloxone (Narcan)
(C) Physostigmine
(D) Ethanol
(E) Diazepam (Valium)
(F) Histamine

491. Atropine

492. Methotrexate

Questions 493–494

For each of the agents below taken by a nursing mother, select the potential toxicity to the neonate.

(A) Pyridoxine deficiency
(B) Kernicterus
(C) Suppression of thyroid function
(D) Staining of developing teeth
(E) Sedation
(F) Ethanol

493. Sulfonamides

494. Propylthiouracil

Questions 495–496

For each patient, select the drug or agent most likely to cause the toxic effect.

(A) Aluminum
(B) Bismuth
(C) Carbon monoxide
(D) Dapsone
(E) Methanol
(F) Gentamicin
(G) Lead
(H) Metronidazole
(I) Nalidixic acid
(J) Primaquine
(K) Ethylene glycol
(L) Sulfamethoxazole
(M) Sulfasalazine

495. A 49-year-old woman is treated for an *E. coli* urinary tract infection. During treatment the woman experiences hemolysis.

496. A 3-year-old boy consumed a liquid from a container in the family garage. He shows central nervous system depression, acidosis, suppressed respiration, and oxalate crystals in the urine. Beside supportive and corrective measures, ethanol was administered to the child.

Questions 497–498

Certain drugs carry a risk of fetal abnormalities if administered during pregnancy. Match each abnormality with the correct drug.

(A) Penicillamine
(B) Diethylstilbestrol
(C) Prednisone
(D) Chloramphenicol
(E) Phenobarbital
(F) Disulfiram
(G) Ethanol
(H) Heroin
(I) Metronidazole
(J) Chlorambucil

497. Malformations of the genitourinary tract

498. Cutis laxa

Questions 499–500

Death from acute poisoning usually occurs by mechanisms that involve vital systems such as respiration, circulation, or the central nervous system. Match each clinical picture with the causative agent.

(A) Cocaine
(B) Carbon monoxide
(C) Strychnine
(D) Atropine
(E) Phenobarbital
(F) Heroin
(G) Phencyclidine
(H) Aspirin
(I) Cyanide
(J) Lysergic acid diethylamide (LSD)

499. Hallucinations, delirium, and coma along with tachycardia and hypertension; hot, dry skin; urinary retention; and dilated pupils

500. Confusion, lethargy, and seizures; hyperventilation and hyperthermia; anion gap metabolic acidosis with dehydration and potassium loss

Toxicology
Answers

475. The answer is C. *(Gilman, 8/e, pp 1632–1633. Katzung, 6/e, p 298.)* Strychnine acts as a competitive antagonist of glycine, the predominant postsynaptic inhibitory transmitter in the brain and spinal cord. The fatal adult dose is 50 to 100 mg. Persons poisoned by strychnine suffer convulsions that progress to full tetanic convulsions. Because the diaphragm and thoracic muscles are fully contracted, the patient cannot breathe. Hypoxia eventually causes medullary paralysis and death. Control of the convulsions and respiratory support are the immediate objectives of therapy. Diazepam may be preferred to a barbiturate in controlling the convulsions because it offers less concomitant respiratory depression. Poisoning caused by the other drugs listed in the question is not associated with convulsions but with depression of the central nervous system.

476. The answer is A. *(DiPalma, 4/e, p 53. Gilman, 8/e, pp 18–20.)* Sodium bicarbonate is excreted principally in the urine and alkalinizes it. Increasing urinary pH interferes with the passive renal tubular reabsorption of organic acids (such as aspirin and phenobarbital) by increasing the ionic form of the drug in the tubular filtrate. This would increase their excretion. Excretion of organic bases (such as amphetamine, cocaine, phencyclidine, and morphine) would be enhanced by acidifying the urine.

477. The answer is B. *(DiPalma, 4/e, pp 161–162, 259, 360. Gilman, 8/e, p 122.)* The organophosphorus insecticides inactivate cholinesterases, which results in accumulation of endogenous acetylcholine in nerve tissue and effector organs. Very severe cases of acute poisoning should be treated first with atropine followed immediately by intravenous pralidoxime (2-PAM). Atropine inhibits the actions of acetylcholine at muscarinic cholinergic receptors, whereas 2-PAM reactivates the inactivated cholinesterases. The effectiveness of 2-PAM in reversing cholinesterase inhibition depends upon early treatment inasmuch as the "aged" inhibited enzyme cannot be reactivated. Diethyldithiocarbamic acid is the active biotransformation product of disulfiram, which is an irreversible inhibitor of aldehyde dehydrogenase. *N*-Acetylcysteine is an antidote used in the treatment of acetaminophen overdosage to prevent hepatotoxicities. Carbachol is a cholinomimetic drug and ethylenediaminetetraacetic acid (EDTA) is a chelating agent. These compounds have no therapeutic value in the treatment of organophosphate poisoning.

478. The answer is B. *(DiPalma, 4/e, pp 357, 360, 413, 748. Gilman, 8/e, pp 657–658, 852.)* Hepatic necrosis can occur with overdosage of acetaminophen. The hepatic toxicity is the result of the biotransformation of acetaminophen to *N*-acetylbenzoquinoneimine, which reacts with hepatic proteins and glutathione. This metabolite depletes glutathione stores and produces necrosis. The administration of *N*-acetylcysteine restores hepatic concentrations of glutathione and reduces the potential hepatotoxicity. Sulindac is biotransformed to sulindac sulfide, the active form of the drug. Both sulindac and its metabolites are excreted in the urine and in the feces. Indomethacin undergoes a demethylation reaction and an *N*-deacylation reaction. The parent compound and its metabolites are mainly excreted in the urine. Procainamide is converted to an active metabolite by an acetylation reaction. The product that is formed is *N*-acetylprocainamide (NAPA). In addition, procainamide is hydrolyzed by amidases. An *N*-acetylation reaction occurs also in the biotransformation of isoniazid. In the liver the enzyme *N*-acetyl transferase converts isoniazid to acetyl-isoniazid.

479. The answer is B. *(DiPalma, 4/e, pp 360, 509–510, 831–834. Gilman, 8/e, pp 1607–1612.)* The chelation agent edetate disodium (Na_2EDTA) causes hypocalcemic tetany on rapid intravenous administration. This effect of edetate disodium is not observed on slow infusion (15 mg/min) since extracirculatory stores are available to prevent a significant reduction in plasma calcium levels. When edetate calcium disodium is given intravenously, hypocalcemia does not develop even when large doses are required. Edetate calcium disodium is used in the diagnosis and treatment of lead intoxication. Edetate disodium is used to treat acute hypercalcemia. The other drugs listed do not cause hypocalcemia. Dimercaprol (BAL) forms chelation complexes between its sulfhydryl groups and metals and is used in the treatment of arsenic and mercury poisoning as well as in certain cases of lead poisoning in children. Penicillamine is the drug of choice in treating Wilson's disease. The agent is also used in the therapy of copper, mercury, and lead poisoning. *N*-Acetylcysteine is an antidote used in the treatment of overdosage with acetaminophen to prevent hepatoxicity.

480. The answer is E. *(DiPalma, 4/e, p 239. Gilman, 8/e, pp 301–305.)* Induction of anesthesia by parenteral administration of thiopental sodium (Pentothal) and other barbiturates is absolutely contraindicated in patients who have acute intermittent porphyria. These patients have a defect in regulation of δ-aminolevulinic acid synthetase; thus, administration of a barbiturate that increases this enzyme may cause a dangerous increase in levels of porphyrins. Administration of a barbiturate would exacerbate the symptoms of gastrointestinal and neurologic disturbances, cause extensive demyelination of peripheral and cranial nerves, and could lead to death.

481. The answer is D. *(DiPalma, 4/e, pp 77–82. Katzung, 6/e, pp 931–942.)* Drug interactions may be beneficial or more often may lead to increased incidences of adverse or toxic effects. Aspirin and other salicylates may increase the hypoprothrombinemic effect of dicumarol. This is because aspirin inhibits platelet aggregation, has a hypoprothrombinemic effect, and displaces dicumarol from plasma proteins. Amphetamines should not be combined with thyroid hormones (e.g., levothyroxine) for weight reduction since the combination can lead to palpitations, increased heart rate, and even cardiac tachyarrhythmias. Cholestyramine would not enhance the effects of acetaminophen. Cholestyramine reduces the oral absorption of acetaminophen and several other drugs, and this reduces the plasma concentrations. Benztropine, a muscarinic blocking agent used in the treatment of parkinsonism, would increase the risk of anticholinergic adverse effects associated with phenothiazines (e.g., thioridazine). Amitriptyline possesses a sedative effect. In combination with ethanol, amitriptyline enhances the central depressant properties of ethanol.

482. The answer is E. *(DiPalma, 4/e, pp 826–827. Gilman, 8/e, pp 801–804.)* Arsenic is an active constituent of fungicides, herbicides, and pesticides. Symptoms of acute toxicity include tightness in the throat, difficulty in swallowing, and stomach pains. Projectile vomiting and severe diarrhea can lead to hypovolemic shock and death. Chronic poisoning may cause peripheral neuritis, anemia, skin keratosis, and capillary dilation leading to hypotension. Dimercaprol is the primary agent used in the treatment of arsenic poisoning. Gingivitis, stomatitis, and salivation are symptoms associated with acute mercury poisoning.

483. The answer is C. *(DiPalma, 4/e, pp 829–830. Gilman, 8/e, pp 1605–1606.)* The liver appears to be spared in cadmium intoxication. Not so the kidney, which in chronic exposure develops proteinuria with extensive damage to the proximal tubule. The symptoms of acute exposure to cadmium fumes are substernal discomfort, myalgias, headache, fatigue, and vomiting. These may be followed in severe cases by wheezing, hemoptysis, and pulmonary edema. In certain parts of Japan, where cadmium industrial waste is common, a syndrome of osteomalacia and bone deformities accompanied by pain and waddling gait is known as *itai-itai* (ouch-ouch).

484. The answer is D. *(DiPalma, 4/e, pp 288, 807. Gilman, 8/e, p 58.)* Activated charcoal, a fine, black powder with a high adsorptive capacity, is considered to be a highly valuable agent in the treatment of many kinds of drug poisoning. Drugs that are well adsorbed by activated charcoal include primaquine, propoxyphene, dextroamphetamine, chlorpheniramine, phenobarbital, carbamazepine, digoxin, and aspirin. Mineral acids, alkalines, tolbutamide, and other drugs that are insoluble in acidic aqueous solution are not well adsorbed. Charcoal also does not bind cyanide, lithium, or iron.

485. The answer is D. *(DiPalma, 4/e, p 260. Gilman, 8/e, p 624.)* Acute intoxication with methanol is common in chronic alcoholics. Headache, vertigo, vomiting, abdominal pain, dyspnea, blurred vision, and hyperemia of the optic disc can occur. Visual disturbances are caused by damage of retinal cells and the optic nerve by methanol metabolites. Severe cases of intoxication can lead to blindness. Other symptoms include bradycardia, prolonged coma, seizures, acidosis, and death by respiratory depression. Since methanol is biotransformed by alcohol dehydrogenase to highly toxic products (formaldehyde and formic acid), ethanol, which has high affinity for the enzyme, is useful in therapy because it reduces the biotransformation of methanol. Other treatments include hemodialysis to enhance removal of methanol and its products and alkalinization to reverse metabolic acidosis. 4-Methyl-prazole, an inhibitor of alcohol dehydrogenase, has also been proposed for treatment. Treatment with ascorbic acid would aggravate the acidosis.

486. The answer is A. *(DiPalma, 4/e, pp 259–260. Gilman, 8/e, pp 378–379.)* Disulfiram is a pharmacologic adjunct in the treatment of alcoholism. When given to a person who has consumed ethanol, it produces flushing, headache, nausea, vomiting, sweating, hypotension, and confusion. The mechanism involves inhibition of aldehyde dehydrogenase; thus acetaldehyde accumulates as a result of ethanol metabolism. Many other agents produce disulfiram-like reactions when administered with ethanol, though their mechanisms have not been established; these include cephalosporins (cefoperazine, cefoperazone, moxalactam), phentolamine, metronidazole, and the sulfonylureas (e.g., acetohexamide and tolbutamide). The tricyclic antidepressant amitriptyline causes sedation. The interaction between ethanol and amitriptyline produces an enhancement of the central depressant properties of ethanol.

487. The answer is E. *(DiPalma, 4/e, pp 811–813. Gilman, 8/e, pp 1618–1620.)* Carbon monoxide is a common cause of accidental and suicidal poisoning. Its affinity for hemoglobin is 250 times greater than that of oxygen. It therefore binds to hemoglobin and reduces the oxygen-carrying capacity of blood. The symptoms of poisoning are due to tissue hypoxia and progress from headache and fatigue to confusion, syncope, tachycardia, coma, convulsions, shock, respiratory depression, and cardiovascular collapse. Carboxyhemoglobin levels below 15 percent rarely produce symptoms; above 40 percent symptoms become severe. Treatment includes establishment of an airway, supportive therapy, and administration of 100% oxygen. It is the cyanide ion that binds to ferricytochrome oxidase and impairs cellular oxygen use, which leads to histotoxic hypoxia.

488. The answer is D. *(DiPalma, 4/e, pp 828–829.)* Unlike lead, mercury, and bismuth poisoning, chronic zinc poisoning does not manifest itself by central nervous system involvement. It can cause anemia and thrombocytopenia. Pancreatic involvement causes a decrease in secretion of amylase. Fever is a common symptom.

489–490. The answers are 489-C, 490-B. *(DiPalma, 4/e, pp 588, 606, 618, 742. Katzung, 6/e, p 895.)* There are many drugs that can produce significant adverse effects on the fetus when given to a pregnant woman. Among these are diethylstilbestrol, which has been shown to produce vaginal adenocarcinoma in female offspring. The incidence of clear-cell vaginal and cervical adenocarcinoma in women exposed to estrogens in utero has been estimated at 0.01 to 0.1 percent. Methimazole may cause hypothyroidism and congenital goiter by reducing thyroid hormone synthesis. Testosterone and derivatives can produce masculinization of the female fetus. Owing to low levels of glucuronyl transferase in the fetus, chloramphenicol increases the risk of gray baby syndrome. Sulfonylurea derivatives, e.g., chlorpropamide, can cause prolonged hypoglycemia in the neonate by stimulating excessive insulin secretion.

491–492. The answers are 491-C, 492-A. *(DiPalma, 4/e, p 156. Katzung, 6/e, p 840.)* The peripheral and central nervous system effects of atropine poisoning may be reversed with physostigmine. Because physostigmine is biotransformed more rapidly than atropine, repeated doses may be necessary. Neostigmine and other quaternary anticholinesterase drugs that do not cross the blood-brain barrier cannot be used to treat the central nervous system effects of atropine.

Naloxone is a competitive antagonist at opioid receptors and is therefore useful in treating overdose with opioid drugs (e.g., morphine, heroin). Because of its short duration of action, repeated doses are usually necessary.

Methotrexate inhibits dihydrofolate reductase and limits the supply of N^5-formyltetrahydrofolate, which is required in the synthesis of thymidylate. Leucovorin (citrovorum factor of N^5-formyltetrahydrofolate) can reduce the toxic effects of methotrexate. Methotrexate therapy followed by leucovorin is a chemotherapeutic regimen for some neoplastic disorders.

493–494. The answers are 493-B, 494-C. *(DiPalma, 4/e, pp 588, 738. Katzung, 6/e, pp 852–859.)* Many drugs taken by nursing mothers can be detected in breast milk. Though some agents (e.g., ampicillin, acetaminophen) have minimal effects, many agents prove to be potentially dangerous.

Sulfonamides have been found in breast milk of nursing mothers. The compounds are highly protein-bound and thus compete with bilirubin for binding to plasma albumin. The higher levels of free bilirubin increase the risk of kernicterus.

Tetracyclines concentrate in breast milk and may cause permanent tooth staining in the infant by binding to calcium. From midpregnancy to 4 to 6 months after birth is the period of greatest danger for deciduous anterior teeth. From 6 months to 5 years of age is the most dangerous period for the permanent anterior teeth.

Propylthiouracil, an agent useful in treatment of hyperthyroidism, can concentrate in breast milk of nursing mothers. The drug significantly suppresses thyroid function in the infant.

Isoniazid reaches rapid equilibrium between breast milk and maternal blood. It can cause pyridoxine deficiency if the mother or child does not receive supplementation.

Central nervous system depressants, such as diazepam or barbiturates, can cause significant sedation in nursing infants.

495–496. The answers are 495-L, 496-K. *(DiPalma, 4/e, pp 260–261, 738, 755, 779, 821–824. Gilman, 8/e, pp 1052, 1055–1056, 1159–1160, 1593–1598.)* Sulfonamides can cause acute hemolytic anemia. In some patients it may be related to a sensitization phenomenon and in other patients the hemolysis is due to a glucose-6-phosphate dehydrogenase deficiency. Sulfamethoxazole alone or in combination with trimethoprim is used to treat urinary tract infections. The sulfonamide sulfasalazine is employed in the treatment of ulcerative colitis. Dapsone, a drug used in the treatment of leprosy, and primaquine, an antimalarial agent, can produce hemolysis, particularly in patients with a glucose-6-phosphate dehydrogenase deficiency.

Ethylene glycol, an industrial solvent and an antifreeze compound, is involved in accidental and intentional poisonings. This compound is initially oxidized by alcohol dehydrogenase and then further biotransformed to oxalic acid and other products. Oxalate crystals are found in various tissues of the body and are excreted by the kidney. Deposition of oxalate crystals in the kidney causes renal toxicity. Ethylene glycol is also a central nervous system depressant. In cases of ethylene glycol poisoning, ethanol is administered to reduce the first step in the biotransformation of ethylene glycol and, thereby, prevent the formation of oxalate and other products.

Lead poisoning in children is most often caused by the ingestion of paint chips that contain lead. Older housing units and homes were painted with lead compounds that produced various colors. Chronic lead intoxication causes such symptoms as basophilic stippling, increased δ-aminolevulinic aciduria, tremors, weakness of extensor muscles, constipation, lead line, and colic.

497–498. The answers are 497-J, 498-A. *(Katzung, 6/e, p 855.)* Practically every drug has warnings concerning administration during pregnancy. Most warn of the increased risk of deformities of limb development and defects like cleft palate. A few drugs carry the risk of distinct organ defects. For example, chlorambucil may cause agenesis of the fetal kidneys. Penicillamine seems to affect fetal connective tissue, causing relaxation of the skin, hypotonia, and hyperflexion of the hips and shoulders.

499–500. The answers are 499-D, 500-H. *(DiPalma, 4/e, pp 166–167, 352–353. Katzung, 6/e, p 845.)* Atropine blocks muscarinic cholinergic transmission in the brain and in the autonomic nervous system. The result is dry mouth, thirst, dry and hot skin, tachycardia, urinary retention, ataxia, restlessness, excitement, and hallucinations followed by stupor, delirium, respiratory depression, coma, and death.

Salicylate or aspirin overdose is characterized by tinnitus, confusion, rapid pulse rate, and increased respiration. The decreased P_{CO_2} plus increased fixed acids at first cause alkalosis which is followed by metabolic acidosis and dehydration and loss of fixed bases. The picture may resemble diabetic acidosis, but the history of salicylate ingestion and blood salicylate levels above 540 mg/100 mL clinch the diagnosis.

Bibliography

AMA Drug Evaluations Annual, 1993. Chicago, American Medical Association, 1994.

DiPalma JR, DiGregorio GJ, Barbieri EJ, Ferko AP: *Basic Pharmacology in Medicine,* 4/e. West Chester, PA, Medical Surveillance, 1994.

Gilman AG, et al (eds): *The Pharmacological Basis of Therapeutics,* 8/e. New York, McGraw-Hill, 1990.

Katzung BG: *Basic and Clinical Pharmacology,* 6/e. East Norwalk, CT, Appleton & Lange, 1995.

Isselbacher KJ, et al (eds): *Harrison's Principles of Internal Medicine,* 13/e. New York, McGraw-Hill, 1994.